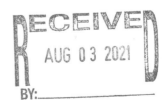

The Brain
on Youth Sports

The Brain
on Youth Sports

The Science, the Myths, and the Future

Julie M. Stamm, PhD

ROWMAN & LITTLEFIELD
Lanham • Boulder • New York • London

This book represents reference material only. It is not intended as a medical manual, and the data presented here are meant to assist the reader in making informed choices regarding wellness. This book is not a replacement for treatment(s) that the reader's personal physician may have suggested. If the reader believes he or she is experiencing a medical issue, professional medical help is recommended. Mention of particular products, companies, or authorities in this book does not entail endorsement by the publisher or author.

Published by Rowman & Littlefield
An imprint of The Rowman & Littlefield Publishing Group, Inc.
4501 Forbes Boulevard, Suite 200, Lanham, Maryland 20706
https://rowman.com

6 Tinworth Street, London SE11 5AL, United Kingdom

British Library Cataloguing in Publication Information Available

Library of Congress Cataloging-in-Publication Data

Names: Stamm, Julie M., 1987– author.
Title: The brain on youth sports : the science, the myths, and the future / Julie M. Stamm, PhD.
Description: Lanham : Rowman & Littlefield, [2021] | Includes bibliographical references and index.
Identifiers: LCCN 2020058417 (print) | LCCN 2020058418 (ebook) | ISBN 9781538143193 (cloth) | ISBN 9781538143209 (epub)
Subjects: LCSH: Brain—Wounds and injuries. | Brain—Concussion. | Sports injuries in children. | Sports—Safety measures.
Classification: LCC RC394.C7 S73 2021 (print) | LCC RC394.C7 (ebook) | DDC 617.4/81044—dc23
LC record available at https://lccn.loc.gov/2020058417
LC ebook record available at https://lccn.loc.gov/2020058418

Contents

Preface

Why I Wrote This Book

This is a book about kids and the consequences of hitting their heads repeatedly while playing contact sports. Sports are ingrained in our culture, making this a controversial topic. I have never played organized tackle football, hockey, rugby, or any other collision sport, but I have spent a great deal of my life around sports, first as a fan, then in a medical role, and later as a researcher. Before we get into the science, I want to tell you why I wrote this book.

I have been a fan of sports for as long as I can remember. My family watched Wisconsin Badger football and basketball religiously. Though I lived in Packer country, I joined a friend on the Miami Dolphins bandwagon. It was the Dan Marino era, and they were in the playoffs consistently throughout my childhood. I was thrilled in 2001 when they drafted both Jamar Fletcher and Chris Chambers, who had been stars for my Wisconsin Badgers.

I'm not just a fan; I'm an athlete. Growing up as a three-sport athlete in a small town in central Wisconsin, sports were my life. Nights were filled with practices or games. Weekends were consumed by tournaments, camps, or open gyms. I played little league baseball with the boys, then softball when a league formed in my town. I joined the volleyball team in middle school, and I still play today. From a young age, basketball was my greatest passion. We didn't travel much, but parents drove me four hours one way to Chicago for basketball camp in the summers. It was a chance to play with some of the best competition in the Midwest, including Candace Parker, one of the best to ever play the game. My junior year of high school we reached the state tournament. This is a big deal in Wisconsin, with local and state media coverage and games airing on television statewide. The entire community rallied behind our team, and we felt like celebrities for a few weeks in our small town.

I chose to attend the University of Wisconsin–Madison over playing a sport at a smaller college, but my love for sports still carried me through my undergraduate years. I began as an intern in strength and conditioning as a freshman. I was a shy, small-town girl working with NHL-drafted hockey players who had just won a national championship. It was intimidating, but this experience gave me confidence and intangible skills that I've carried with me through life.

I became a student in the athletic training program my junior year, and my first clinical rotation was with the Badger football team. I learned a lot about sports medicine while providing care to the football players. You see almost any type of injury in football, from lacerations to fractures to concussions and everything in between. I also learned a lot about the football environment: the culture, the athletes, the attention, and the daily grind.

I had clinical rotations with a variety of other sports at the University of Wisconsin, and I worked with many incredible athletes. Some went on to be stars in professional leagues, and some became Olympians. Yet the athlete that had the greatest impact on my life and career was a young high school football player. One day he came into the athletic training room saying he just didn't feel right after a hit in practice. Nothing was overly concerning on his exam, and we determined that he had what I would have called at that time a mild concussion. But unlike most concussions, this athlete's symptoms lingered for months. He was just out there playing a sport with his friends. Yet he suffered an injury that significantly altered his life, impacting his academics, social life, and ability to live a normal day. It was such a heartbreaking scene to watch unfold, and it plays out all too often in young athletes.

This case sparked my drive to study concussions and their consequences on the young brain. I moved to Boston and spent a year as a graduate assistant athletic trainer, learning from the incredible staff at Boston University. I met Dr. Robert Stern, director of clinical research at the Chronic Traumatic Encephalopathy (CTE) Center at Boston University, and, with some persistence (a skill I learned through sports), found my way in as an intern there. I earned a spot in a PhD program in anatomy and neurobiology the following year and became dedicated full-time to studying CTE and the long-term consequences of concussions and repetitive subconcussive impacts in sports. I focused my dissertation research on the consequences of repetitive hits to the head during childhood, when the brain is still developing. The findings of that research are one reason I am writing this book.

Why am I telling you all of this? Because I want you to know that I get it. I understand the importance of playing sports. Like so many other people, sports are a big part of my story. I am an avid sports fan and athlete from a small town who become a neuroscientist, anatomist, and researcher. Athletics have played an immeasurable role in making me the woman I am and helped me develop so many of the qualities that have allowed me to be successful: leadership skills, work ethic, grit, determination, teamwork, and more. The skills and qualities I developed in the venue of sports were critical to get me where I am today.

Some people feel the researchers studying brain trauma in sports are out of touch with the sporting world. They think we don't understand the game, the culture, or what it means to be so invested in a sport. While I believe this is true in a few cases, it is simply not the truth most of the time. It's definitely not true of the researchers I worked with at the Boston University CTE Center. Many of us are athletes, and all are passionate sports fans. It's part of why we care so much about keeping athletes safe and healthy. I get the importance of sports, including football, to so many children and adults both in this country and around the world. But I have also seen what some sports have done to those who dedicated part of their lives to the game.

I still want to be a football fan, although I am finding the game harder and harder to watch—even my beloved Wisconsin Badgers. I used to have games on TV all day on Sundays. I would plan my Saturdays around the Badger game. But now, though I still watch sometimes, it isn't the same; I know too much about what happens inside the helmet.

This truly makes me sad. A part of my life that I really enjoyed is gone. *I want to be a fan*, but knowing what I know now, I feel guilty watching and supporting the sport in its current state. I know there are people out there who feel the same way. And it's not just football. Other sports like rugby, soccer, and hockey are facing similar challenges. I hope that, with some significant changes, we can all enjoy watching—and playing—these sports again.

Sports participation has so many incredible benefits to millions of youth athletes. I learned this firsthand. My experience as an athlete had an enormous positive impact on my life. Kids need to have the opportunity to play sports, and they should be able to do so without the risk of permanently damaging their brains. That is why I wrote this book.

Part I

Youth Sports: The Wins and the Losses

Throughout this book, I will refer to these sports in the following way:

Football—American football
Soccer—what is called "association football" outside the United States
Australian football—Australian football
Hockey—ice hockey
Rugby—rugby union, rugby league, and rugby sevens, unless specified

When I refer to contact sports in this book, I am referring to collision and contact sports that expose athletes to repetitive impacts and brain trauma. Some contact sports, like basketball, do not expose players to repetitive brain trauma. However, I will group the contact and collision sports above as "contact sports" for simplicity.

If I am discussing a non-contact or limited-contact form of football, I will specify flag, TackleBar, or flex football. If only "football" is referenced, it is referring to tackle football.

Chapter One

Why We Should Care about Repetitive Brain Trauma in Youth Sports

The fact that we are knowingly subjecting 5-year-olds to a brain disease
will baffle anthropologists for centuries to come.

—Chris Borland, former NFL player[1]

I start every presentation I give on the consequences of repetitive brain
trauma in youth sports with a seven-second video from a youth football
practice.[2] The athletes in this video are about eight or nine years old.
Two players are in an athletic crouch, facing each other, and sur-
rounded by their teammates and coaches. The coach blows a whistle,
and the two young athletes run toward each other full speed. A bystand-
er yells, "Go! Go!" They lower their heads and deliver a crushing blow
with the tops of their helmets. In the background, the crowd lets out an
"oooooh" at the sight of the brutal hit. One player stands up quickly and
walks away. The other young boy curls up into the fetal position on the
grass, moaning and crying.

You don't have to be a doctor or a neuroscientist, or know anything
about the brain, to recognize that what happens in this video *can't* be
good for a child (or anyone, for that matter). Luckily, these drills are
banned in many leagues now, but similar collisions still happen in the
game today. These hits put children at high risk of not only brain injury
but also devastating spinal cord injury. Impacts to the top of the head

send force through the head and neck that can shatter vertebrae and leave the athlete paralyzed.

As hard as these hits are to watch, they aren't the only ones that are concerning. Repetitive blows to the head, like those sustained by linemen on every football play or with every soccer header, can change the brain, even over a single season. When these hits happen in childhood, while the brain is rapidly developing, the consequences can be even greater. Kids may be smaller, but routine impacts cause forces to their brain similar to those experienced by high school and college athletes. [3] And they can experience hundreds of impacts in just one season.

You don't even need to hit your head to damage your brain. A blow to the body can cause a whiplash effect that transmits forces to the brain. Have you ever watched a replay of a tackle that caused a concussion and thought, "That didn't look like a bad hit"? It might not have been, but if the head moved with enough force in the right way, even if it wasn't touched, it can stretch and strain the nerve cells, or neurons, in the brain.

Whether you're a sports fan or not, you have probably heard something in recent years about brain trauma in college and professional sports. But the majority of athletes never reach those levels. How many young athletes are exposed to repetitive brain trauma in youth contact sports each year?

- *Hockey:* Over 380,000 athletes ages eighteen and younger played hockey in the United States in the 2017–2018 season. [4] Around a half million youth players are registered with Hockey Canada, [5] and there are over 1.1 million players around the world under age twenty. [6]
- *Soccer:* Soccer is enormously popular worldwide, with over 21.5 million players under age eighteen. [7] In the United States, nearly seven million children under age seventeen play soccer annually, with around two-thirds of those being under age twelve. [8]
- *Rugby:* Rugby is a growing sport worldwide. More than 2.2 million youth athletes played the game in 2018 alone. [9]
- *Lacrosse:* The popularity of lacrosse is growing in the United States, with over 281,000 children ages six to twelve [10] participating and 210,000 playing at the high school level. [11]
- *Football:* Over one million high school athletes play tackle football annually. [12] An estimated 2.5 million athletes play youth tackle football, including nearly 900,000 between the ages of six and twelve. [13]

Tackle football has the highest risk for repetitive brain trauma as an inherent part of the game. The number of youth and high school athletes in the sport has been declining over the past decade, in part due to these safety concerns. The vast majority of football players haven't reached high school, and the youngest players in some leagues are just five years old.[14] Youth programs often have the least resources, guidance, and safety oversight. Yet their athletes are playing the same game with the same equipment standards and most of the same rules as the bigger, faster, and stronger college and professional players.

Research is still lacking on the short- and long-term consequences of brain trauma in the youngest players. The research that has been done often neglects to consider how sport-related brain trauma interacts with normal childhood brain development. The attention from both the public and science has been on those playing under the bright lights on Friday nights and in the big stadiums on Saturdays and Sundays.

Although it makes sense that hitting your head a lot as a kid is not a good thing to do, there has been some resistance to the idea that it can have significant long-term consequences. Much of this comes from sports culture. I have often heard the excuse, "I played football as a kid and I'm fine." Others "want their kid to learn to be tough!" Football is an American pastime, and other sports like rugby and soccer are treasured aspects of societies around the world. Many fans love the big hits, and they believe some sports wouldn't be the same without them.

Other resistance comes from the research world. In science, we want absolute proof that A causes B before we are willing to accept it. Unfortunately, certainty and proof in science is hard to come by. While it is important to strive for, definitive proof is often unrealistic, incredibly hard to achieve, or could take decades to establish while putting many at risk in the meantime. To prove that exposure to repetitive impacts could alter a child's brain development, we would have to study many children in a controlled environment. They would have to live in the same place, eat the same foods, and do the same activities. Then half of those children would need to be intentionally subjected to repetitive head impacts throughout childhood. Clearly, this completely unethical study will never happen.

A realistic version of this study would follow children throughout their lives, starting before they begin participating in sports. Many years later, we would compare those who played contact sports in childhood and those who didn't. Though a few studies exist that follow children through adulthood, they aren't designed to look at this topic. Most concerning, the answers wouldn't be known for decades. Though this study should still be done, we simply can't wait that long for answers. Too much is at stake.

Some have argued that no major changes should be made to youth sports until we have definitive proof of the connection between repetitive brain trauma in sports and long-term consequences. Yet the public health perspective says we need to make decisions based on the best information we have now to minimize potential risk. As you'll learn in this book, there is growing evidence that experiencing repetitive head impacts over time can have consequences later in life. There is also evidence that repetitive brain trauma in childhood, while the brain is rapidly maturing, could alter typical brain development, leading to lasting consequences. Taken together, there is enough evidence to warrant taking strong precautions to avoid repetitive brain trauma in youth. It's true that we don't know everything, but that doesn't mean we know nothing.

Nearly every day I see news articles about concussions in athletes or chronic traumatic encephalopathy, the degenerative brain disease thought to be caused, in part, by repetitive trauma to the brain. We hear about the decline of some of our favorite sports legends. We hear about depression and suicide in former professional athletes as well as young athletes who never had the chance to become legends. These stories, and the confusing, sometimes conflicting messaging from the scientific community, have left many parents with questions about the potential consequences their children could face from brain trauma in sports.

The conversation around head impacts in sports is often incomplete or inaccurate. New research is frequently misinterpreted, exaggerated, or oversimplified unintentionally in the media or, in some cases, intentionally to fit a desired narrative. For example, a study found that 110 out of 111 NFL players had CTE. Many misinterpreted that to mean 99 percent of football players get the disease.[15] However, the researchers never made any claim about disease prevalence. When a study found that high school football did not lead to later-life cognitive issues, some athletic associations were quick to use this to promote the safety of high school football.[16] Among other issues, the study only included people who played high school football in the 1950s, a time when the game looked very different than today. Other studies have been funded or conducted by leagues or companies with vested interests in the outcomes. In some cases, it is still solid research, but in other cases the conflict of interest combined with questionable study design warrants skepticism.

At the same time, youth sport organizations are touting changes they have made to make their sport safer. Soccer associations have banned or restricted heading at youth levels. American and Canadian hockey organizations and US Lacrosse have banned checking at young ages. These changes have been aimed at reducing injuries and eliminating sources of repetitive brain trauma in these sports.

The loudest voices are often from those involved in tackle football. The sport is woven into the fabric of American culture, so removing an aspect of the game for youth players, even for the sake of children's health, can be a matter of great controversy. Some claim that "proper" tackling techniques, new concussion education initiatives, and high-tech helmets have made the game "safer than ever." Youth football organizations, state athletic associations, and the NFL have gone to great lengths to convince parents, especially moms, that the game is safe for their kids.[17] Calls to ban tackling at youth levels have been met with protest, despite support from NFL stars. The sport has made many changes throughout its history to calm the fears of parents and fans. But is it really "safer than ever"? Is "safer than ever" safe enough?

With any public health issue, the passion driving differing viewpoints often leads to a war of words in which the commonalities between both sides are lost. I love sports and think all kids should have the opportunity to play, but I do not believe it is in the best interest of children's long-term health to experience unnecessary brain trauma in the pursuit of those sports. In the end, we all want to reach the same goal: an atmosphere where children can compete in the sports they love, learn life lessons, make friends, and do so *safely*.

Families need accurate, unbiased information so they can make informed decisions. Health care providers need to understand the research so they can have appropriate answers for parents. Coaches need to know what they can do to keep their athletes safe. This book will break down the science, explain what we actually know and what we have yet to learn about repetitive brain trauma in sports, and provide guidance for families and others involved in youth sports.

Chapter Two

How Youth Sports Can Provide a Lifetime of Benefits

> Sports is the greatest metaphor we have for life, teaching you things like how to deal with anxiety, how to deal with communicating with each other, leadership, performing under pressure. All those are valuable lessons.
>
> —Kobe Bryant, eighteen-time NBA All-Star [1]

Before we dive into the dangers of repetitive brain trauma in sport, I want to talk about the *importance* of sports. Sports can have an immensely positive impact on a child's physical and mental health and help children develop essential life skills, including discipline, dedication, and teamwork. This is above and beyond the benefits of physical activity alone.

Unfortunately, participation in many youth sports in the United States, and around the world, has declined in recent years. In some sports this decline has been blamed, in part, on concerns about brain injuries and their potential long-term consequences. Concerns about brain health are valid, but they shouldn't be a reason to quit sports altogether.

This chapter will give context to why it is so important that we do everything we can to protect children's brains while preserving their opportunities to play sports. This issue is far bigger than one sport or one team. The decline in participation and calls to ban certain sports entirely are incredibly concerning. This has implications for the health and well-being of our country and world for years to come.

PHYSICAL AND MENTAL HEALTH BENEFITS OF PLAYING SPORTS

Playing a sport provides wonderful opportunities to have fun while being physically active. Physical activity has countless benefits for our health and well-being. Even a single session of moderate or vigorous physical activity can have immediate health benefits, such as reducing blood pressure and improving insulin sensitivity.

Many health benefits of youth sport participation stem from preventing obesity. Obesity in youth has been linked with type 2 diabetes, fatty liver disease, anxiety, depression, high blood pressure, and early signs of heart disease, among other conditions.[2] Physical activity in sport is more important than ever, as the prevalence of obesity grows around the globe. More than one-third of children are overweight or obese. The United States has the highest childhood obesity rate in the developed world. From 1980 to 2014, obesity rates have more than doubled in children and quadrupled in teenagers. Obese children are likely to grow up to be obese adults, and obese parents are far more likely to raise obese children, perpetuating the cycle of obesity.

The health consequences of childhood obesity also linger into adulthood, even if the individual reaches a healthy adult weight. Adults are at higher risk of suffering heart attacks or dying from coronary heart disease if they were obese as children.[3] The risk of type 2 diabetes, hypertension, kidney issues, and cancer are also higher in adults who were obese in their youth.

Participation in team sports can help children and adolescents get physical activity and maintain a healthy weight, especially if they play more than one sport.[4] But it's not quite that simple. The Centers for Disease Control and Prevention (CDC) recommends that children and adolescents between the ages of six and seventeen should do at least sixty minutes of moderate to vigorous physical activity each day.[5] Moderate activity makes your heart beat a little faster than normal, including activities like biking or walking at a somewhat fast pace. Vigorous activity increases your heart rate and breathing rate even more with activities like jogging, a hard bike ride, or running or jumping in sports. Kids should be involved in a variety of activities that build muscle and bone strength, develop different motor patterns, improve their cardiovascular fitness, and challenge them in different ways. Many youth sports check most or all of these boxes.

Just sixty minutes a day of activity equivalent to walking at a reasonably fast pace shouldn't be that hard for kids to meet, right? Wrong. Only 24 percent of youth meet the CDC recommendations.[6] You might think kids who play sports would have no problem meeting these recommendations, but that's not exactly true either. Children who play organized sports are more likely to reach the recommended physical activity levels on days that they play compared to children who don't play a sport, but that doesn't mean that all, or even most, do.[7]

Imagine a child has practice for their favorite sport one Saturday. If the practice is ninety minutes, it's logical to think they must hit their daily physical activity goal. Unfortunately, that's likely not the case. You may be surprised to learn that only a quarter to half of practice time, in this example, about twenty-five to forty-five minutes, is spent doing activity at moderate to vigorous levels.[8] Up to half of practice time can be spent standing in line, waiting for a turn, or watching a demonstration. Most practice drills aren't intense enough to raise an athlete's heart rate high enough and long enough to see health benefits, and game participation might not be enough to reach those levels either.

The sport played makes a difference. Research has shown that soccer, competitive or recreational, tends to provide the greatest amount of physical activity. Participation in soccer as well as basketball, track and field, and other sports have been associated with reduced weight in kids and teens. On the other hand, children playing sports like baseball, softball, and football, which involve intermittent bursts of activity, are less likely to reach their physical activity goals.[9] Many young tackle football players are hitting their heads repeatedly without gaining the health benefits of physical activity thought to be associated with the sport (more on that later). Playing sports is a step in the right direction toward reaping the health benefits of physical activity. When enough moderate and vigorous activity is intentionally incorporated in practices, the results can be tremendously beneficial for the health of young athletes.

The mental health benefits of playing sports extend far beyond those that come from physical activity alone. Students who participate in youth and high school sports tend to have better self-esteem, self-image, self-knowledge, emotional regulation, and overall quality of life than nonathletes.[10] Most athletes are also at lower risk of emotional stress, anxiety, depression, and suicidal behavior. Other activities, like art and music, can have a positive impact on youth too, but research suggests that sports can have even greater benefits for brain health and reduced depression than participation in these other activities.[11]

The social aspect of being on a team amplifies the benefits for young athletes. Children and adolescents develop friendships and form strong bonds with teammates.[12] Coaches may be mentors or even parental figures for kids. The sense of support and belonging, feelings of acceptance, and the ability to lean on teammates for success contribute to reduced depression and anxiety in athletes.[13] In a nationwide study of children ages nine to eleven, involvement in team sports was related to the volume of a brain structure called the hippocampus.[14] This structure plays a critical role in forming new memories, and a smaller hippocampus has been associated with depression. The larger hippocampal volume observed in only team-sport athletes was associated with reduced depression in boys. These results support the idea that being part of a team has even greater effects on the brain than exercise alone.

Participating in sports can lead to improved cognition and higher academic achievement. Better physical fitness and endurance are associated with better integrity of the pathways connecting brain regions and improvements in memory, processing speed, problem-solving, planning, concentration, impulse control, and other cognitive functions.[15] Fit children are better able to take in new information, analyze that information, and use it right away, and they are more likely to earn better grades than students who are inactive or obese.[16] Playing a high school sport can encourage student-athletes to attend class, earn good grades, go to college, and have higher professional aspirations.[17] As you can see, sports without repetitive impacts are actually really good for the brain!

SPORTS PROVIDE EXTRAORDINARY OPPORTUNITIES TO LEARN LIFE SKILLS

Any athlete, coach, or parent of an athlete will likely tell you that playing sports can be a great way to develop life skills. Athletes need to coordinate, communicate, and resolve conflicts with teammates and coaches. They need to be accountable for their actions, disciplined, willing to sacrifice, and put in the work and effort to improve for the team. They learn to work toward a common goal and follow through on the necessary steps to achieve that goal. They also learn to control emotions in stressful situations, persevere through challenges, and cope when things don't go their way. Student-athletes have to manage their time to successfully balance schoolwork, sports, family commitments, and sometimes work responsibilities. These skills are key to being successful in many aspects of life.

This isn't just hearsay or personal opinion; this is supported by science. For example, research has shown that participation in sports can help athletes improve their decision-making and problem-solving skills.[18] Youth athletes tend to work better with others and form stronger peer relationships than youth who do not play sports. Participation in sports is also associated with greater empathy and honesty, following rules, and supporting and encouraging others.

Of course, the sport setting isn't the only place where children and adolescents can learn life skills, and the messaging shouldn't be conveyed that way. Likewise, no single sport is superior or the only sport where these skills can be learned. Still, sport participation offers many great opportunities to learn many skills necessary for success in life outside of sports: at school, in the community, at work, in social settings, at home, and beyond. This is, of course, one of the many reasons we should fight to keep organized sport opportunities while also protecting our children's developing brains. These don't have to be separate goals.

THE BENEFITS OF CHILDHOOD SPORTS PARTICIPATION LAST A LIFETIME

Childhood and adolescence are critical times for developing fitness habits that last. Playing sports as a child increases the likelihood that a person will be physically active through adulthood. In one study, those who participated in organized sports at age ten were more likely to do regular physical activity at age forty-two.[19] The same was not true for those who only reported regular outdoor play at age ten. This means participation in sports may have a greater influence on the durability of habits created in childhood, making them more likely to persist for a lifetime.

This is a big deal. The CDC estimates that a lack of physical activity is the root cause of around 10 percent of premature deaths and $117

billion in health care costs each year.[20] Physical activity recommendations drop to only 150 minutes of moderate activity each week in adulthood. Yet only about a quarter of adults hit that mark.

Other benefits from sports translate into adulthood as well. Youth
and high school athletes are more likely to play varsity or recreational
team sports in college, and college students who participate in team
sports at any level report lower depression scores.[21] Participation in
high school sports has been linked to higher career attainment and
taking on higher-level leadership roles in adulthood.[22] Sports can be a
great way to gain life skills that carry into the workforce.

CONSIDER THE IMPORTANCE OF SPORTS

Unquestionably, playing sports can benefit youth in many facets of life.
When discussing changes to improve safety in sports, completely banning certain sports for kids should not be part of the conversation.
Changing contact sports to eliminate the greatest sources of repetitive
brain trauma, at least at young ages, is a far better option. These
changes could encourage more kids to play some sports, as has been the
case with hockey,[23] and bringing more kids into sports allows those
kids to reap the many benefits sports have to offer.

Chapter Three

Why Sports Culture Needs
a Transformation

The game sets up the wrong kind of hero—the man who uses his
strength brutally, with a reckless disregard both of the injuries he may
suffer and of the injuries he may inflict on others. That is not the best
kind of courage or the best kind of hero.
                                        —Harvard President Charles Elliot, 1894 [1]

In 1961, Albert Bandura ran an experiment in his laboratory that involved an inflatable clown named Bobo. One group of children
watched an adult play quietly, largely ignoring Bobo. Another group of
children watched an adult take out aggression on Bobo, throwing, kick-
ing, and even hitting the clown with a hammer. When the children had
their chance to play, those in the first group played gently with Bobo.
But the group that watched the aggressive adults mimicked that behavior, pummeling the poor clown. This experiment demonstrated Bandura's social learning theory: children learn behaviors from observing
others around them. [2]

The social learning theory holds fast in the sports world. Kids see
World Cup soccer players collide going for a header, then hear the fans
cheer as a player stands up, her face bloody, and continues playing.
They see their rugby coach demean another player for being "weak"
and missing a tackle, and they take that language home to yell at their
brother. Kids see the star football player lower their helmet to lay a
crushing hit on their opponent, and they think hitting their opponent

like that will show their own toughness. A study found that fights occurred in nearly a third of hockey games.[3] This wasn't at the NHL level. This was in pee-wee hockey with eleven- to twelve-year-old players. They aren't even allowed to check until age thirteen, but these players said that they felt that fighting was just part of the game. Young athletes see this behavior from the stars they idolize, and they imitate it.

These behaviors are part of a culture developed and molded through the history of sports. This culture holds toughness among the most important and admirable traits of an athlete regardless of the consequences it imposes on athletes themselves. Many children start playing organized sports by age five or six. Their indoctrination into this culture can start that early too, with attitudes and behaviors being reinforced not only in every practice and game they participate in but also every time they watch their favorite teams play.

This chapter will discuss the culture of sports and how it affects the attitudes and behaviors of athletes when it comes to brain safety. Sports culture reveres players who sacrifice for the team. If athletes act in the best interest of their health, it may be seen as a sign of weakness or a lack of dedication. This is one reason most concussions go undiagnosed and players continue to put themselves at risk.

THE CULTURE OF SAFETY IN SPORTS (OR LACK THEREOF)

An athlete's perception of the culture of safety in sports is shaped not only by their own values and beliefs but also by the influence of parents, coaches, teammates, the community, the media, and more.[4] When weighing all relevant factors in any situation, it is common for safety to be considered, but ultimately placed low on the priority list, in part due to the expectations or behaviors of others. In the workplace, employees may be less likely to report injuries or safety concerns due to fear of losing pay, being treated differently by their boss or colleagues, or losing their job.[5] Similarly, on any given play, athletes have to weigh their own safety against the potential to make a play that will help the team win, the chance to impress recruiters, potential criticism for simply protecting themselves, and more.

Optimism bias is also a factor. We don't think something bad is going to happen to us, so we are more willing to take risks. Even when athletes are informed of the risks repeatedly by coaches, medical providers, or others, they often continue to use risky tactics. In a survey of high school football players in Hawaii,[6] about 80 percent said they used their helmet to hit an opponent, with nearly half saying they did it intentionally and nearly 30 percent saying they did it more than ten times in the previous year. All players, by law, had received concussion education. Nearly all reported that they knew they could hurt themselves, and three-quarters knew that they could hurt another player. Yet optimism bias prevails. Athletes often think concussions won't happen to them. If a concussion does happen in sports, it's in situations that are out of their control, or freak accidents. Many don't believe their behavior plays a role in the injury.

If athletes know that dangerous plays like targeting in football or boarding in hockey could cause serious injury to them or their opponent, why do they do it? Because it's sports culture. Inflicting pain on the opponent draws cheers from the crowds. A willingness to inflict pain on oneself for the sake of the team makes a player a hero. For a devoted athlete, the ability to play through pain can be as important as proper footwork or learning the plays. Bruises are a source of pride if they are the result of hustle and sacrifice.

A willingness to sacrifice for the sake of the team can be a beautiful thing. There are special bonds formed as a result of experiencing stressful and intense sports moments together, fighting to achieve a common goal. The toughness and willingness to sacrifice learned on the field can help us overcome challenges in life off the field. But the idea of what it means to be tough can be taken too far. For example, athletes sometimes play through significant injuries, like broken bones, torn ligaments, and concussions, to stay in the game. Defensive back Ronnie Lott even had part of his finger amputated to avoid the long recovery he would have had with surgery to repair the broken finger.[7]

Both the highest sports leagues and the media glorify the culture of toughness and playing through pain. For years the media had segments highlighting the biggest hits of the week. Broadcasters can say little about brain trauma in sports without facing backlash. Bob Costas was pulled from the Super Bowl broadcast in 2019, supposedly due to comments he made at a journalism symposium about the league's denial of science showing that trauma from football damages the brain.[8] If he had a twelve- or thirteen-year-old son, he said he would not let him play tackle football. NBC let this happen to Costas because they didn't want to lose the chance to air NFL games. The league could simply break ties with any network for saying too much about brain trauma in football, and the network would be out substantial money. Networks have to stick to the messaging about the heroism and toughness of the athletes.

The mentality that an athlete protecting themselves is a sign of weakness or lack of dedication to the team can also be reinforced by fans. In 1959, Montreal Canadiens goaltender Jacques Plante took a puck to the face.[9] Before he went back into the game, he demanded to wear the fiberglass face protection that he typically wore in practice. Fans questioned his bravery, toughness, and loyalty because he insisted on wearing the mask. Today we couldn't imagine watching a hockey game with a goalie who wasn't wearing a mask.

Fans have become accustomed to the violence, the injuries, and the pain. In some sports it can be easy to forget that there is a person inside the helmet. When you can't see their face, it's easier to ignore that the pain and damage is being inflicted on another human being for the sake of entertainment. Researchers at Auburn University conducted MRIs on football fans and nonfans.[10] They showed each participant violent images of football collisions and violent images unrelated to football. The nonfans reacted the same way to the violent images no matter what the source of the violence was. The football fans had a different reaction. Areas of the brain involved in empathy and the perception of pain were activated in their brains when they saw the violent images unrelated to football, but those regions were not activated when they saw violent football images. The fans may have been desensitized to the violence when it was in the football setting. These findings would likely apply to other sports too.

All of this builds a culture that says a player's health doesn't matter, as long as they do what it takes to help the team win. Most fans don't know that, after all of the sacrifice, players are often left out to dry. The average NFL career lasts only 3.3 years, but players have to be in the league for four seasons to get health care when their career is over. Even those who played for a decade or more only get health care for five years after retirement. After that, they are on the hook for surgeries or therapy they need as a result of the trauma of their playing days. It's similar at the college level. Once the athlete graduates, they no longer receive medical care or coverage for lingering injuries. Some don't even get insurance coverage for injuries while they're in school. Most universities and professional leagues do little to support retired athletes after they profit from the abuse of their bodies and brains.[11]

Fans idolize the legends who are great at their game, but they are really idolizing the legend over the person. Few people ever see what many legends become after their time in the game has ended. It seems like a normal thing for a child to idolize a sports superstar, but what if being a superstar makes it difficult to function in daily life in middle age? What if being a superstar changes their personality and mind in a way that takes a substantial toll on their family? What if being a superstar gives them a brain disease? Is that what our kids should be striving for?

THE SPORTS CULTURE CAN ENCOURAGE ATHLETES TO HIDE CONCUSSIONS

Most athletes don't like to talk about concussions, repetitive impacts, or the potential long-term consequences of brain trauma. When they do, they often downplay risks or say it's just part of the game. They are afraid they will look soft or scared. There is no place in the battle for weakness, and reporting concussion symptoms may be interpreted by many as just that.

Most states, universities, and athletic organizations require athletes to receive concussion education.[12] Unfortunately, knowledge doesn't always translate into improved attitudes or behavior. The invisible nature of concussions means they are easy for athletes to hide. In most cases, if the athlete doesn't disclose their symptoms, it's hard for coaches or medical staff to know that the athlete has a concussion. If a player feels "dazed" after an impact, they shake it off and move on to the next play like they do with other injuries. If coaches ask if they are okay after a hit, athletes often simply say yes and keep playing. While concussion reporting has improved in recent years, we still have a long way to go.

Research has shown that between one-third and more than three-quarters of athletes don't report concussion symptoms.[13] In 2013, my colleague Dr. Christine Baugh surveyed more than seven hundred college football players from ten schools around the country.[14] She asked about their diagnosed concussions and the times that they had concussion symptoms but didn't report them to their coach or athletic trainer. For every one diagnosed concussion in their career, the athletes had an average of four concussions they didn't report. They also reported having a "ding" or getting their "bell rung" over nineteen times for every one diagnosed concussion, with linemen reporting these symptoms most often. The average player knowingly continued to play with concussion symptoms nearly seven times in their football career.

Athletes have given many reasons for why they choose to hide their concussion symptoms, including the following: [15]

- They didn't know they had a concussion or that the injury was serious enough.
- They weren't aware of the potential consequences of playing through a concussion.
- They didn't want to come out of the game.
- They were afraid they would look weak.
- They were afraid of letting their teammates or coaches down.
- They felt pressure from teammates, coaches, parents, or other fans to continue to play.
- They were concerned about losing playing time or their position on the team.
- They were afraid of ending their career or losing their scholarship. (The majority of college scholarships are one-year contracts and not guaranteed for four years. A scholarship can be pulled if a player is injured.) [16]

The first two reasons have to do with a lack of knowledge, but educational efforts have led to some improvements in recent years. Seventy percent of girls' soccer players in one study continued to play with symptoms before legislation mandating concussion education was passed. [17] After the legislation passed, 54 percent reported playing with concussion symptoms. Yet the fact that over half of girls' soccer players would still play while symptomatic is quite concerning, and it shows that simply giving athletes knowledge is not enough.

The willingness to report concussion symptoms seems to be more related to the athlete's attitude about concussions and sports, concerns about what will happen if they report the injury, and cultural norms within the team or sport than to their concussion knowledge. [18] Athletes who believe they will receive criticism or negative consequences, whether from coaches, parents, teammates, or fans, are less likely to report their injury. At least a quarter of college athletes have been pressured by at least one of these groups to keep playing when they had a concussion. [19] If pressure comes from multiple directions, athletes are even less likely to disclose their injury

Several studies have found that males are less likely to report their concussion symptoms than females. The masculine culture of toughness in sports plays a role. Male athletes are more likely to report that teammates and coaches would be angry with them or think they were weak or less masculine if they disclosed the injury.[20] Females may be more likely to take the injury seriously, and that could make them more likely to report. However, this trend isn't true across the board. Female college athletes in one study had greater intentions to report, but there was no difference between males and females in the actual likelihood that they would keep playing with concussion symptoms.[21] In another study, youth girls' soccer players were five times more likely to continue playing with a concussion compared to boys.[22]

Some athletes are afraid that other players will think less of them for reporting the injury. In one study, youth athletes said they thought their teammates would be upset if they left the game because they had a concussion.[23] Over 90 percent of community-level rugby players understood that playing with a concussion was dangerous, but nearly a third said they would keep playing even if they had symptoms.[24] Four in ten said they felt they would be letting their teammates down if they reported their concussion symptoms and stopped playing in the game. Not surprisingly, if a championship game was on the line, up to half of athletes have reported that they would play with concussion symptoms.[25]

Coaches play a critical role in forming the culture of their team. The attitudes and behaviors displayed by coaches around concussions influence the willingness of their athletes to report. Athletes may feel more pressure to continue playing with a concussion if their coach has ridiculed them or given negative feedback for reporting injuries in the past. Coaches control playing time, and if the coach feels an athlete is weak or unwilling to sacrifice for the team, they may be less likely to play. Some coaches make statements about athletes simply being a number, concussions not being as serious as a broken leg, or not believing that an athlete has symptoms.[26] Even if the coach doesn't explicitly tell their athletes not to report, the culture of safety (or lack thereof) that they create, and their overall attitudes toward injured players, can give the perception, real or not, that the coach would not support the athlete in reporting their concussion. In contrast, athletes who feel the coach supports them in reporting their concussion symptoms are more likely to follow the right protocols if they suspect they have a concussion.[27]

Research has shown that most coaches today view concussions as serious injuries and understand that they have a responsibility to remove athletes from play if they suspect a concussion. However, similar to athletes, when the importance of the game increased, the likelihood that the coach would remove the player from the game decreased. While 92 percent of coaches would remove the athlete from a regular season game, only 83 percent said they would remove a concussed athlete from a championship game.[28]

When coaches create a culture that puts their athletes at risk, they rarely see the repercussions. They can encourage their athletes to do whatever it takes to win, even if it puts them at risk, but when the athlete is injured, they put in the next man up. Coaches may praise athletes for big hits, but when the same type of hit results in an injury, it is simply "bad luck" and the coach takes no blame. This culture isn't just responsible for brain injuries. It can also lead to other life-threatening conditions from training intended to toughen athletes up, such as heat stroke and rhabdomyolysis (a potentially deadly condition involving muscle breakdown from overexertion). Toughening athletes up can come at the greatest cost for the athlete, whether immediately or decades later. Yet there is often little or no cost for the coach.

The weight a person gives to their athletic identity can influence their behaviors around safety in sports. For some players, their whole identity and most of their daily activities revolve around being an athlete. In one study, male college hockey players with strong athletic identities were less likely to report their concussion.[29] If their identity is strongly tied to their participation in sports, they may be willing to risk both their short- and long-term health to stay in the game.

That athletic identity can also extend to the athlete's family. Many families consider themselves to be "sports families." In an interview study with parents of middle school football players in Texas, several parents discussed how football was a central part of their identity as a family.[30] It filled their conversations and much of their time. Their involvement in the sport was vitally important to their family, and there was never a question of whether or not their child would play. In some cases, parents forced their child to play football, even if they weren't interested in the sport. The risks of football were not concerning to the "football families." Parents sometimes pressured athletic trainers and coaches not to pull their children from games due to a concussion, despite knowing the risks of continuing to play.

Parent attitudes about concussions influence their children's attitudes and willingness to report symptoms. Nearly one-quarter of youth rugby players surveyed felt that their parents would want them to keep playing if they sustained a potentially concussive head impact.[31] Parents who put more pressure on their child to succeed are less likely to promote concussion reporting, and their children are less likely to report symptoms. Some parents are concerned that reporting a concussion will make their child miss opportunities.[32] In contrast, parents who have positive attitudes toward concussion safety may discuss the injury with their kids, including the importance of reporting the injury for their health and how it can help the athlete perform better in their sport. This increases the likelihood that their child will report concussion symptoms.

Sports and community are undeniably intertwined. Football games are a major social event. A growing number of high schools have multimillion-dollar stadiums that seat ten thousand or more fans. Even parents who are highly concerned about the safety of football for their own child enjoy spending their Friday nights watching other people's kids collide on the gridiron. Children see the high school athletes as superstars, and they see the way the community reveres them. Understandably, kids want to experience the glory too.

Community support can also have a dark side. Community influence can make parents feel as if they have no control over whether or not their child participates in contact sports. Of course, parents are fully capable of making that decision for their child, but it's not easy to go against pressure from friends, family, coaches, or other members of the community. Youth athletes and their parents have been ridiculed by friends and even family members for choosing an alternative to tackle football.[33] Some coaches will go around parents and talk to the kids themselves, encouraging them to play. This is especially true for kids who are athletic or large in stature because coaches think the child will help the team. Sometimes parents go directly to the kids too. At a youth football game, I witnessed the mother of a player on the team trying to convince an eleven-year-old boy that he should play. She did this right in front of the boy's mother, who she knew was holding him out of the sport at his age out of concerns for his safety. An adult woman pressuring a child to act against his mother's wishes is absurd, but it happens all too often in the world of youth sports.

Kids can have a lot of fun playing non-contact versions of football or rugby. Yet they may be labeled soft or weak by coaches or other members of the community. But in all honesty, if a kid can only have fun in sports if he or she is crushing another kid with a big hit, shouldn't we be a little concerned?

THE NEED FOR A CHANGE IN SPORTS CULTURE

Cultural norms can be incredibly hard to change. When those attitudes and behaviors become part of our lives at a young age, shifting those norms later can be an insurmountable task, even if they are putting kids in harm's way. Children watch their idols exemplify the culture of sport in every game. By the time some children reach high school, they may have been part of this culture for nearly a decade. It's all they know. This culture of toughness, playing through pain, and not wanting to appear weak has led some to hide concussion symptoms, despite the knowledge of the potential consequences of doing so. In addition to concussions, other repetitive head impacts take their toll too. Sports culture tells athletes that taking so many of those hits makes them appear tougher and more willing to sacrifice for the team.

The culture of sports has also become a culture of denial when it comes to brain trauma. Athletes deny that they have concussions in part because they deny that the injury is serious, or they worry a coach will deny them playing time or a position on the team. Professional leagues deny any negligence or liability, saying that the athletes knew their sport could damage their brain. But this is only after denying, some-times for decades, that the game carries that much risk to begin with. The culture of denial is critical to the survival of contact sports as they are today.

The denial even extends as far as discrediting solid science. Let me be clear: One study is never the be-all and end-all of a topic. Every study has limitations, and every good research paper clearly lays out those limitations. No science is perfect. That's why we need many studies to shape our knowledge on a topic. This does not mean that any one study is useless on its own. A study can be very suggestive of something even when we still need more research. Our understanding is shaped and reshaped with each new study that comes out. When new study findings contradict previous results, it doesn't necessarily mean the first study was wrong. It just adds to the story. Yet the culture of denial has tried to say that not knowing everything means we know nothing. The constant evolution of science makes it easy for some to deny any danger.

In the next part of this book, I will discuss what we do know about the science, and what we still have to learn. It's true that the science is far from complete, but what we know thus far is compelling. Yet without a change in the culture of sports, the science alone may do little to keep our athletes safe.

Part II

The Science: What We Know about Repetitive Brain Trauma in Sports

Chapter Four

Why Kids Really Do Hit That Hard

Exposure data shows children as young as nine are getting hit in the head more than 500 times in one season of youth tackle football. That should not feel normal to us. Think of the last time, outside of sports, you allowed your child to get hit hard in the head twenty-five times in a day.

—Chris Nowinski, cofounder and CEO of the Concussion
Legacy Foundation[1]

One Saturday morning I attended a sixth-grade football game with a friend. I was talking with a mother about head impacts in the sport when a player's father turned around and said, "They're just kids, they don't hit that hard."

This is a common misconception I hear from parents and coaches alike when I talk about head impacts in youth contact sports. They believe the smaller, slower players can't possibly hit that often or sustain impacts hard enough to affect the brain like older, stronger, faster players. It seems logical. The hits don't look that bad. Kids aren't tackling with the speed and ferocity of NFL or National Rugby League players. They aren't entering open-ice collisions at NHL speeds. They aren't vying for headers like the US Women's National Soccer Team. It would make sense that youth athletes wouldn't incur the same kind of trauma to the brain that the adults do.

Unfortunately, that isn't quite true. A child's head grows rapidly in youth, making it disproportionately large compared to the rest of their body. This essentially makes a child somewhat like a bobblehead doll.[2]

Their weak necks have a harder time stabilizing their head, causing it to more easily whip around with any hit or a fall to the ground. Add the weight of a helmet and the situation is even worse.

Our understanding of the number and magnitude of impacts experienced by athletes of all levels has grown immensely in recent decades. This chapter will describe technology that allows us to measure these hits and what we have learned about the number and magnitude of hits sustained by youth athletes compared to their older and more experienced counterparts. As you will see, they aren't all that different.

HOW ARE HEAD IMPACTS MEASURED?

I want to start by explaining how head impacts are measured in sports. Keep in mind that, although we often use the term "head impacts," researchers aren't just measuring the impacts directly to the head. They are measuring how the head moves. A blow to the body or falls to the ground can cause rapid head movements, a whiplash-like effect that can strain and damage the brain, even though the head was never actually touched.

Special sensors, called accelerometers, are used to measure acceleration of an impact.[3] Higher acceleration translates to greater force experienced by the athlete from the impact. The sensors also provide the total number of hits that exceed a minimum threshold of force. Why have a minimum threshold? Because every movement results in some degree of acceleration on our brain, but not all of these forces are dangerous. The minimum threshold helps to ensure the accelerations measured by the sensors are actually from impacts and not due to other movements like running or jumping.

Accelerometers provide information about both linear and rotational acceleration of the head. Linear acceleration, measured in g-force, is essentially the strength of a head acceleration in one direction.[4] If a player takes a 100 g impact, the impact is 100 times the force of gravity on that player. Even if the player isn't moving very fast, the abruptness of a collision can lead to big head accelerations. Common activities, including walking, running, and jumping, typically fall under 6 g.[5] Most studies in the field use a minimum threshold between 10 and 15 g to exclude these incidental forces.

Rotational acceleration occurs along a rotational path around an axis, like a spinning top.[6] Rotational forces can occur when you turn your head quickly from right to left or experience a whiplash effect from front to back or side to side, for example. Concussions are usually caused by a combination of linear and rotational acceleration, but rotational acceleration may be even more damaging due to the strain the brain is under as it twists and hits against prominent structures inside the skull.[7] Boxers often target the mandible, or lower jawbone, when trying to knock out their opponent because a blow to that area can cause high rotational forces.[8]

In sports like hockey and football, accelerometers can be placed in the helmet. For nonhelmeted sports, companies have developed mouth guards or skin patches with accelerometers. The sensors transmit data wirelessly to a computer or device on the sidelines. No sensors are perfect, but mouth guard and patch sensors tend to have higher error rates than helmet systems, more often counting impacts that didn't happen. Video analysis is typically used to verify impacts in research. Some companies are selling accelerometer systems commercially, claiming they can help to recognize concussions or track impacts. I will discuss these sensors in chapter 10.

HOW MANY HITS DO ATHLETES SUSTAIN PLAYING THEIR SPORT?

Research using accelerometers has given us valuable insight to what a typical practice, game, or season of impacts looks like in various sports and at different playing positions. I will focus more on football in this section simply because more research has been conducted on football players. However, in recent years, we have learned more about the impacts sustained by athletes in other contact sports too.

Football is one of the most popular sports in America. It can also deal its players hundreds of impacts over the course of the average season. Both college and high school players average between 300 to 775 head impacts in just one season and nine to fifteen impacts per event, which includes practices and games.[9] It is common for some players to experience over one thousand hits in a single season. The average high school season has sixty-five to seventy events over a few months of time. Shockingly, in just one season, one high school player sustained 2,235 impacts,[10] while a college football player sustained 2,492 impacts.[11] In one study, a football player experienced 108 impacts on a single day.[12]

But those are older athletes. What about kids in youth football? Most research shows youth athletes ages nine to fourteen sustain an average of two to three hundred head impacts above 10 g in one season.[13] Several studies had a number of players incur more than five hundred, or even eight hundred, impacts. A youth season typically includes fewer than half the events of a high school or college season, so the overall number will be a bit lower. Yet, similar to the high school and college players, youth players experience an average of eight to sixteen impacts per event. At the high end, an athlete in one study sustained 1,226 impacts in one youth season, while another experienced fifty-four impacts in a single event.[14]

Even the youngest players, those ages six to nine, incur an average of 110 to 160 impacts per season (typically about fifteen events) and six to eleven impacts per event. Some young players experience many more impacts than that. One eight-year-old player sustained 374 impacts in thirteen events, for an average of twenty-nine impacts per event.[15]

Those defending youth tackle football have cited a 2014 study of twelve- to thirteen-year-old players suggesting that kids playing Pop Warner football only sustain an average of sixty impacts each season.[16] Let's be clear, there is no evidence that sixty head impacts over several weeks is safe for kids. Aside from that, the study used a sensor system with a 30 g minimum threshold, compared to the 10 or 15 g threshold in most other studies, which means they likely missed a substantial number of impacts sustained by the youth players. It also only included six games and five practices, notably less than youth seasons in most other studies. One of the study authors, who is also the chairman of Pop Warner's Medical Advisory Committee, referred to these findings when discussing youth football safety in the media.[17] The organization would benefit from parents feeling comfortable with the current safety of youth football. But how are parents, guardians, or coaches supposed to fully understand the risk when the only information they are getting from a national youth football organization uses data from a study designed markedly differently than the rest of the field? No study is without limitations, but honesty about limitations and how a study compares to other similar research is key for those making decisions that affect a child's safety.

Two studies have examined impacts in flag football. In one study, youth and high school athletes experienced an average of 0.1 head impacts per player for every ten minutes of seven-on-seven flag football play.[18] A conservative estimate from other research suggests about two head impacts occur per tackle football player in the same time frame. Head impacts increased slightly with age in flag football but still remained low. No head-to-head contact occurred in the flag football players in this study—the head impacts were primarily head to ground or head against another player's body while attempting to catch a pass. In another study, youth tackle football players experienced nearly five times more impacts than youth flag football players per event, including seven times more impacts in games.[19] The flag football players only sustained about one impact for every two events. This evidence suggests that head impacts are *far* less frequent in flag football than tackle football.

While the number of impacts sustained by youth tackle football players tends to be lower over shorter youth seasons, the average number of impacts per practice or game are not far off from older players. Kids can still experience hundreds of hits in just one season, with some athletes sustaining numbers that well exceed the average impacts over a high school or college season. Far fewer impacts occur in flag football, though, and playing this version of the game in youth could greatly reduce the cumulative burden of impacts an athlete experiences over their playing career.

How do head impacts in football compare to other sports? Male high-school- and college-age hockey players experience an average of 280 to nearly 500 impacts over a season, with maximum numbers ranging from 446 to 785.[20] Female hockey players are not allowed to check at any level, yet they still average around 170–230 impacts per season. Overall, hockey players average between three to eight impacts per event. At the youth hockey level, boys sustain around 140–225 impacts per season, while one study found girls sustained only around thirteen per season.[21] We still have much to learn about hockey impacts, particularly for female players and those under age thirteen.

In soccer, heading the ball is the most obvious cause of repetitive head impacts, but head-to-head impacts while attempting a header and head-to-ground impacts when falling are also common. High school and college soccer players experience approximately two to seven head impacts per event and fifty-five to 160 per season at the college level, far less than hockey and football.[22] A study conducted in the early 2000s, long before rules were implemented banning or limiting heading in youth programs, found that youth soccer players ages ten to thirteen years old headed the ball an average of 186 times and up to 450 times over about sixty events.[23]

A few studies have looked at other sports. Youth rugby players in the under-eleven and under-nine age groups sustain an average of thirteen and ten impacts per match, respectively.[24] The average youth Australian football player in one study sustained about five impacts per game.[25] College men's lacrosse players experience between three and twelve impacts per event, while high school girl's lacrosse players sustain an average of just two impacts greater than 20 g per season.[26] Overall, there is a substantial gap that needs to be filled with data on these sports at the youth level.

HOW POWERFUL ARE THE HEAD IMPACTS ATHLETES EXPERIENCE?

Now let's address the misconception that "they're just kids, they don't hit that hard." In football, the average linear acceleration for impacts in high school and college is around 20 to 29 g, and the average rotational acceleration ranges from around 1200 to 1700 rad/s^2.[27] What does this actually feel like? A force of about 25 g is comparable to that felt by a person crashing their car into a wall at thirty miles per hour.[28] This is just the average though. Any football fan knows that big hits are part of the game. Hundreds of impacts exceeding 60 g can occur on a team each season, and several even exceed 100 g. The maximum accelerations in one study were 205.3 g linear and 10,484 rad/s^2 rotational,[29] nearly double that of a hard punch thrown by an Olympic boxer.[30]

You may be surprised to learn that the average force of impact at the youth level is similar to that of their college and high school counterparts.[31] Across studies of nine- to fourteen-year-old tackle football players, the linear acceleration from most hits fell between 18 and 25 g, and rotational acceleration ranged from 850 to 1400 rad/s^2. Players aged six- to nine-years-old sustained hits with a slightly lower average force, usually between 15 and 18 g. In most youth football studies, about one in twenty impacts exceeded 50 g, and several hits in each study exceeded 80 g. The highest linear acceleration experienced in each study ranged from 100 to 179 g. Even seven- to eight-year-old kids were capable of generating a hit with a linear acceleration of 111 g. These are extraordinary numbers that absolutely show even the youngest tackle football players are capable of experiencing high-acceleration impacts.

Football isn't the only sport that can deliver high-force impacts. Most impacts in men's and women's hockey range from 15 to 31 g at the college and high school levels.[32] Around 85 percent of youth hockey impacts have a linear acceleration below 30 g. However, like football, accelerations in youth hockey can exceed 100 g.[33]

Most soccer impacts at the college level are between 15 and 25 g, while impacts at the youth level tend to have a linear acceleration around 18 g. Though far less frequent, several hits over 50 g do occur in soccer, with the highest recorded hit in one study being 115 g.[34] In a youth soccer study, male players sustained more head impacts than female players, but the female players were more likely to experience high-magnitude impacts.[35]

Data is lacking at the youth level in other contact sports. Though a few studies show youth rugby and Australian football players experience average impacts around 15 g,[36] we need more research to understand the force of impacts on these athletes.

WHAT FACTORS INFLUENCE HEAD IMPACT EXPOSURE IN SPORTS?

Several factors influence the number of impacts an athlete sustains. These factors are important to understand because they can be targets of interventions aimed at decreasing repetitive brain trauma in sports.

Player Position: In most contact sports, the number and force of impacts can vary greatly by the position the athlete plays. This is most evident in football. Offensive and defensive linemen consistently sustain the most impacts of any position on the field.[37] Every play, with the exception of a kickoff, involves linemen crashing into each other at the line of scrimmage. It is common for linemen to experience more than a thousand impacts, or even two thousand impacts, in just one season. These hits tend to be of lower accelerations compared to players at other positions. They don't have time to gain much speed before they collide with each other. Players at the "skill" positions tend to sustain fewer overall hits but more hits at higher accelerations than linemen because they have more space to generate speed before impacting their opponent. Multiple studies have suggested that, on average, running backs sustain the greatest number of high-acceleration hits. Despite the fact that quarterbacks are often protected in practice, a season at this position can lead to more than three hundred head impacts.

Most players competing in high-level college football play only one position on either the offensive or defensive side of the ball. At the high school level, though, it is more common for an athlete to play both offense and defense. One player might play both wide receiver and cornerback, for example, while another might play both offensive and defensive lineman. Playing on both sides of the ball leaves the athlete vulnerable to taking significantly more hits in a season.

Positional differences occur in other sports too. College midfielders in soccer tend to sustain the most impacts over a season, averaging more than ninety-five impacts, while goalies average just ten impacts.[38] In youth hockey, defenders tend to experience slightly more impacts than forwards, and again, goalies experience the fewest impacts.[39]

Event Type and Timing: The intensity of the game setting tends to lead to a greater number of overall impacts and high-magnitude impacts. Yet, because there are far more practices than games, practices contribute the most to the overall number of hits over a season.[40] Preseason can be a time for players to prove their skills and value to the team, and preseason practices tend to have more impacts than in-season practices.[41]

Type of Play: Across sports, certain plays leave athletes vulnerable to high-level impacts. A greater starting distance between players means they can gain more speed before hitting each other. In football, this is most common on kickoffs, punts, and passing plays.[42] This is one reason for rule changes regarding the kickoff across all levels of football play over the last decade. Plays in which infractions, or penalties, occur can also result in more severe impacts. A youth hockey study found illegal plays resulted in higher linear and rotational accelerations not just for the person being hit but also for the player who delivered the hit. Rule enforcement can play a critical role in keeping players safe.

Awareness of the Oncoming Hit: Tackles, checks, or other contact from behind or outside the view of the impacted player are more likely to result in high-acceleration impacts compared to impacts a player can anticipate.[43] In soccer, for example, purposeful headers result in lower accelerations than unanticipated head impacts.[44] When the athlete sees the impact coming, they can tense their body and neck and prepare for it, reducing the impact accelerations.

Experience: More experienced athletes tend to incur more impacts than those who are new to a sport.[45] With more experience, players gain confidence with tackling and hitting, and they may be more willing to engage more aggressively in plays they would have avoided before. More experience may also mean more playing time and more impacts.

Individual Player Attributes: The talent an athlete has and the aggressiveness level he or she plays with can influence the number of impacts they sustain in a season.[46] In a study of youth football players, those who demonstrated greater overall athletic ability generally sustained more head impacts over a season, especially in games, compared to their less-athletic teammates.[47] Those with more athletic ability may reach greater speeds and may be involved in more plays, leaving them more vulnerable.

More athletic and aggressive players may choose to expose themselves to the most headers, check more, or tackle more. Aggressive players may be more likely to use their head as a weapon in helmeted sports, which can lead to more high-acceleration impacts.[48] Some play with a reckless abandon that makes them fantastic athletes but also makes them more likely to endure hundreds or even thousands of head impacts over a season. This isn't just dangerous for that player; one overly aggressive player can increase the risk of injury for other players too.

In a study of hockey players, more aggressive players sustained a greater number of severe impacts, particularly in practice, but had a similar number of overall impacts as less aggressive players.[49] The less aggressive players rose to the intensity of their more aggressive teammates in games, but they knew when to back off in practice to keep themselves and their teammates healthy. The more aggressive players, however, carried those intense hits into practice, too, even though they were inflicting those impacts on their teammates.

Coaching and Team Culture: Coaches dictate many aspects of a team that influence the impacts a player experiences. For example, football coaches determine the style of offense a team runs. In a 2013 study, offensive players in a run-first offensive scheme incurred 50 percent more impacts than those in a pass-first offense over a season.[50] However, the pass-first offense, with more open-field, higher-velocity plays, resulted in players sustaining impacts with higher average accelerations.

Coaches determine the training drills players perform in practice, and in football, tackling drills leave players at substantially higher risk of sustaining impacts over 40 g. Drills such as "king of the circle," "Oklahoma," and "bull in the ring," where players run and hit another player from several yards away, result in the highest force of impact.[51] Fortunately, these drills have been banned by most youth football leagues, though some teams continue to use them to "toughen up" their players. Scrimmages and game-situation drills with open-field plays can also lead to significant impacts. Lower-acceleration impacts are most common with drills focusing on passing and technique. The same goes for other sports. In soccer, coaches control the amount of practice time spent on heading. Tackling drills and scrimmages in rugby as well as hockey and lacrosse drills involving checking and full-speed play can leave those players at risk of a higher number and more severe head impacts.

Coaches influence the culture and attitudes of the team regarding safety, and in turn, they can encourage the aggressive nature of play that some athletes bring to the game. As a result, rules and regulations that simply decrease the time teams are allowed to spend in full-contact practice may not make a substantial difference in the amount of impacts players sustain. Aggressive coaches and players alike will simply pack those hits into a shorter amount of time, making the effect of reducing contact practice time negligible.

WHAT DOES IT ALL MEAN FOR YOUTH ATHLETES?

While the data on head impacts in various sports isn't perfect, it gives us a better sense of the kind of repetitive trauma to the brain athletes sustain on a regular basis. What does this mean for the future of athlete safety? The answer right now is we don't know. Sure, sports can provide many benefits for those who participate, but experiencing that many hits over a few months provides nothing but harm. It is possible that some combination of hits at certain accelerations might increase your risk of sustaining a concussion during a given day, week, or season. It's also possible that the right combination of hits along a spectrum may increase the risk for long-term issues, such as CTE. Maybe fewer hits at a higher magnitude and more hits at a lower magnitude carry similar risk for future impairment or disease. We just don't understand this relationship yet.

Someday it is likely that we will be able to use all of the information we have learned on repetitive brain trauma from accelerometer-based research to make better health decisions for our athletes on an individual basis, perhaps using some kind of hit count, similar to a pitch count in baseball. For now, we still have a lot to learn.

Chapter Five

Why the Young Brain Is Vulnerable

Youngsters, especially between the ages of ten and twelve, are developing connectivity networks. . . . If there is an injury, these pathways are going to be altered, and it can have a significant effect on what the personality of the individual is going to be. He may not have been programmed genetically to wind up with problems with depression or cognitive issues, but that can be the net result.
—Robert Cantu, MD, medical director and director of clinical research, Cantu Concussion Center[1]

To understand the potential consequences of repetitive trauma to the developing brain from the hundreds or even thousands of impacts experienced in youth sports, we have to understand what typical development looks like. Brain development from childhood to young adulthood involves bursts of rapid maturation and an intricate pattern of processes that shape the person we become. These rapid periods of development are also windows during which the brain is most vulnerable to poor outcomes from trauma. This is important to consider when weighing the risks and benefits of contact sports for young athletes. Kids are *not* just little adults.

This chapter will give a brief overview of childhood and adolescent brain development and explain why the brain is so vulnerable during the ages when many kids are playing youth sports. I will share examples of what can happen when development is disrupted in the brain and provide supporting evidence of disrupted development from other environmental causes in the brain and body.

A BRIEF INTRODUCTION TO BRAIN DEVELOPMENT

We are born with nearly all of the neurons we will ever have—more than 100 billion.[2] The most rapid stages of brain growth occur before birth, with an average of 250,000 neurons being created every minute. But after we are born, we make very few new neurons, so if we damage our neurons throughout life, we are not able to replace them.

The brain reaches 90 percent of the size of an adult brain by age six.[3] Clearly, a six-year-old child has a lot of growing to do, and their brain function is far from that of an adult. In fact, brain development and maturation continue well into early adulthood, but overall brain size stays about the same for most of that time. Instead, brain development occurs through the refinement and rearrangement of pathways and connections within specific brain structures.

Myelination is the process of wrapping a fatty sheath around a neuron's axon, the long tail-like structure that carries information from one neuron to another.[4] The fatty layer gives the axon a whitish appearance, so pathways formed by myelinated axons make up the brain's white matter. Due to ongoing myelination, the white matter volume increases from childhood through adulthood. Like the coating around a copper wire, myelin insulates the axon and allows electrical signals to travel more rapidly along it. The more myelin on an axon, the faster the signal speed, even up to 120 meters per second. Though not all neurons have myelin (it depends on a neuron's job), when myelin is present, it is critically important to the function of the neuron.

Children have less myelin than adults. This can be problematic because myelin also helps protect the axon. Axons with little or no myelin are more exposed, making them more prone to damage with concussive and repetitive impacts and the chemical changes that occur in the following hours and days.[5] They also don't recover as well from injury as highly myelinated axons. This means a child's axons are more vulnerable to damage with brain trauma in sports.

Although we make very few new neurons after birth, we do form around 100 trillion new synapses, or connections, between neurons through childhood to allow more information to be shared between different parts of the brain.[6] These synapses are located in the brain's gray matter, along with the cell bodies that control the neuron's function. Synapses take up space, so as we create more connections, our gray matter volume increases.[7] We make synapses at a rapid pace from birth until a given structure reaches its peak in childhood or adolescence. But the brain actually makes too many synapses, which can affect how the brain functions. It's like when two signals are competing for the same radio frequency, so you hear two songs at the same time. Likewise, having too many synapses causes excessive noise in the brain as too many neurons compete to send their signal to the same target. This makes it harder for a child's brain to function efficiently, leading to subtle challenges like slower reaction time.[8]

The brain deals with this noise through a process called synaptic pruning.[9] Imagine if by simply listening to your favorite radio station more, you could eliminate those other weak radio signals interfering with the frequency. With synaptic pruning, the strongest, most-used connections are retained, and the others are eliminated.[10] This loss of synapses is a *good thing* that allows the brain to work better, and it is very different than the loss of connections that occurs with aging or conditions like Alzheimer's disease. As we prune unnecessary synapses, the brain refines the structures and pathways needed to complete a given function.

The pruning process begins shortly after a gray matter structure reaches its peak size and number of synapses, and it results in a decrease in the structure's size over time.[11] This is in large part why the brain doesn't grow very much in size after age six. The exact timing of the peak differs by structure. Areas that process our senses, like vision, peak and begin pruning in early childhood.[12] Other areas, such as those involved in complex functions like planning and reasoning, reach their peak around age twelve but continue pruning into the midtwenties.

Myelination and synaptic pruning allow different parts of the brain to work together more quickly and efficiently.[13] This contributes to better cognitive function and behavior control as children mature. For example, while children are capable of some high-level cognitive functions, they struggle as the task or situation becomes more complex.[14] A child can control their impulses in some situations, but they gain the ability to do so consistently and in a variety of situations as they mature into adulthood. Our experiences in childhood and adolescence play a key role in how our connections are formed and pruned.[15] For example, the brain of a child who is a skilled musician will produce and prune synapses differently than a child who is a star basketball player. These processes also play a role in how our emotions, personalities, and individuality develop.

Brain structures go through specific time windows of rapid development called critical periods.[16] Critical periods can involve surges in synapse formation, rapid rates of myelination, or substantial pruning and refinement of synapses. The timing of critical periods varies in different regions and structures of the brain, and a structure can go through multiple critical periods, with on-off cycles, at different points throughout childhood and adolescence. There seems to be a correlation between some critical periods and the onset of puberty, especially with synapse formation and pruning.[17] In most cases the peak is reached earlier in females than males, as females tend to reach puberty at a younger age.

Several gray matter structures and white matter pathways have a peak developmental stage between ages eight and twelve.[18] The following paragraphs describe the development of a few important structures and processes I will discuss in upcoming chapters.

Corpus Callosum: The largest white matter pathway is the corpus callosum, which allows communication between the right and left sides, or hemispheres, of the brain.[19] It contains up to 250 million axons, and it plays an important role in coordinating attention, language, and other complex cognitive tasks. The corpus callosum has a critical period of rapid myelination between ages eight and twelve, with most of it reaching 90 percent of full myelination by age eleven.[20] This pathway is frequently damaged by concussive trauma and brain trauma from repetitive impacts. As the brain moves and rotates with trauma, one hemisphere hits against supportive tissue within the skull, while the other hemisphere pulls away, stretching and damaging the axons in the corpus callosum as it continues to connect the hemispheres.[21]

Hippocampus: The hippocampus is vital for learning and forming memories. It is a key structure affected in Alzheimer's disease, which is why those with the disease have a hard time remembering new things.[22] This structure reaches peak volume between ages ten and twelve and decreases in size after that as a result of synaptic pruning.[23]

Amygdala: The amygdala plays a key role in processing emotions, understanding social interactions, and regulating fear and anxiety. This structure sees a critical period for connectivity around age ten and reaches its peak volume around age twelve.[24]

Prefrontal Cortex: The cortex is the layer of gray matter along the surface of the brain. Several cortical regions have a wave of growth in late childhood followed by pruning starting around age twelve.[25] The prefrontal cortex, at the front of the brain, is responsible for many of our executive functions, or complex cognitive processes such as multi-tasking, problem solving, planning, inhibiting impulses, and decision making.[26] These skills help us understand a situation, weigh potential responses, and choose the best one. Though the prefrontal cortex reaches a peak in synapses in early adolescence, it continues to remodel well into our twenties.

Metabolism and Blood Flow: Myelination, synapse development, and pruning take a lot of energy. The resting metabolism of the brain, or the amount of fuel the brain uses at rest, is considerably higher in children than in adults.[27] This fuel is carried in our blood, and a peak in blood flow to the brain occurs between ages ten and twelve.

CRITICAL PERIODS AND WINDOWS OF VULNERABILITY

It was once believed that the young brain could handle trauma better than the adult brain because of its plasticity, which is the ability to adapt and reorganize in response to its environment.[28] While plasticity is far more limited in adulthood, scientists thought the young brain could simply reorganize and compensate for brain trauma without consequence because it was still being molded into its adult form. While the developing brain can compensate for some degree of damage, the natural plasticity and development process can be altered by trauma like concussions.[29] Altered plasticity can actually disrupt the ability of other structures to fully develop their intended functions, as they may have to compensate for the damaged structure.

Childhood brain development is like building a house: it has to be built on a solid foundation that will support the floors above.[30] The connections made throughout childhood brain development form a critical foundation for the adult brain. If this foundation is not laid the proper way, it may lead to cognitive, emotional, or other deficits down the line, some more subtle, others more significant. The earlier this damage occurs, the worse the outcome may be because less of the solid foundation has been laid before the process was disrupted.

The brain may be prepared to handle small disturbances and return to the normal path.[31] In this case, a child would reach the expected adult structure and function. But after larger disturbances, the brain can change developmental paths, and the final outcome can differ from the original plan. Effects of a concussion or repetitive impacts could change how synapses are formed or pruned or inhibit normal myelination, altering the brain's developmental trajectory.[32] The adult brain has completed these processes, so the outcomes of brain trauma in childhood can look very different than the outcomes from the same trauma in an adult.

Skills that are not mature yet or that are developing at the time of the injury are most vulnerable.[33] Improvements in executive functions like information processing, impulse control, and attention between ages eight to twelve lay the foundation for gains in strategic thinking, planning, and other executive functions through adolescence. If typical development is disrupted, children can fall behind, resulting in delays in reaching normal function, or perhaps never reaching normal function at all. For example, learning is intended to follow a typical path for children throughout their school years. If executive functions are impaired early, it can result in difficulties learning new, more advanced skills later. A complex algebra problem requires strategic thinking, organization, and planning skills to solve. A typically developing high school student would have the skills needed to learn how to solve the problem. If a student incurred brain trauma several years earlier affecting the development of his executive functions, he may struggle to solve the problem. Such a student may seem to function well overall, but deficits can become apparent with increasingly complex tasks.

Critical periods are a time when the experiences a child or adolescent has, both positive and negative, can have the most influence on brain structure and function.[34] Critical periods can be windows of opportunity in which the brain can positively adapt to experiences.[35] Unfortunately, critical periods can also be windows of vulnerability. Let's say, for example, that a brain structure X undergoes rapid growth from ages eight to ten. If a child is exposed to brain trauma that affects structure X at age six or twelve, the effects may be less severe. However, if the same exposure occurs at age nine, the outcome may be much worse. If disruption occurs during a critical period, it can cause an even greater deviation from the intended path.

Many cognitive difficulties from disrupted brain development have one crucial thing in common: the symptoms don't show until the child is older, even into their early twenties.[36] If language skills are impaired, it is evident in childhood because these skills develop early.[37] But it's hard to know if executive functions, which fully mature by the mid-twenties, have been disrupted in an eight-year-old because those functions are supposed to be limited in children. If that eight-year-old grows up to be a twenty-eight-year-old who continues to struggle with things like planning, impulse control, and decision making, you might think something is wrong. If these skills don't fully develop, the individual is often thought to have personality flaws, be a disorganized person, or have a "short fuse." You likely wouldn't attribute these behaviors to disrupted development that occurred twenty years earlier.

DISRUPTED DEVELOPMENT

There has been some resistance to the idea that repetitive head impacts could damage the brain or alter the way the brain develops. However, this concept is well accepted by medical professionals and scientists regarding other body systems. Normal brain development can be disrupted by a number of outside factors, too, leading to lasting changes in brain structure. The specific age when the exposure occurs influences the outcome. To demonstrate this point, here are a few examples of disrupted development:

Fractures: When a fracture occurs in a child's growing bone, it is well accepted that the growth of that bone may be disrupted or altered. The growth plate is where the bone grows in length. A fracture that damages an active growth plate can cause it to close and stop growing prematurely, resulting in a bone that is shorter than it would have otherwise been.[38] Fractures to the middle of the bone can also alter bone development. As the bone begins to mend, cells that make new bone go into overdrive, resulting in the injured limb being longer than it was meant to be.[39] However, these outcomes would not happen if the fracture occurred in adulthood.

The Developing Lungs and Smoking: Alveoli in our lungs are the balloon-like structures where oxygen and carbon dioxide are exchanged between our blood and the air.[40] We are born with only about one-sixth of our alveoli. We develop more throughout childhood, but growth increases dramatically around the onset of puberty until we peak with at least 300 million alveoli by our early twenties. This makes adolescence a critical period for lung development. Any form of smoking in adolescence can disrupt the development of our alveoli, potentially resulting in a lower peak number of these critical sites of gas exchange and potentially a lower overall lung capacity.[41] Smoking in adolescence also increases the risk of developing lung cancer because lung cells that were altered by smoking replicate as new alveoli develop.[42]

Childhood Obesity: Obesity can also alter the anatomy of a child's heart by causing an increase in the size of the chambers on the left side of the heart, which pumps blood out to the body.[43] These changes in the structure of the heart in childhood and adolescence can persist into adulthood, even in those who reach a healthy weight as an adult.

Radiation Exposure in Children: Those who are exposed to radiation from X-rays and CT scans in childhood are at greater risk of developing cancer, including brain tumors, later in life compared to those not exposed or those exposed in adulthood.[44]

Lead Exposure: Children exposed to even low levels of lead can have significant cognitive impairments, including difficulties with attention, memory, and reaction time.[45] Lead exposure in childhood is also associated with poor academic achievement as well as behavioral challenges, including poor impulse control, withdrawal, delinquency, and social difficulties. These symptoms often don't show at the time of exposure; instead, they appear later in life, when certain skills are supposed to come online but never fully develop. Lead exposure in adulthood, especially at lower levels, does not typically have the same level of consequences.

Alcohol Use: Alcohol is toxic for the developing brain, especially when consumed while binge drinking. This can disrupt myelination, synapse formation, and synaptic pruning.[46] The prefrontal cortex is particularly vulnerable and tends to be thinner in those who consume alcohol regularly in their teen years. Frequent drinking also alters white matter development, resulting in smaller white matter volumes than expected. Functionally, those who start binge drinking in adolescence have a number of cognitive and behavioral issues, including memory issues, a lack of impulse control, and anxiety, that persist into adulthood even if they stop drinking.

Cannabis Use: Adolescent cannabis use has been linked to low academic achievement and difficulties with memory, learning, and other cognitive functions that last into adulthood.[47] Altered cortical thickness and disrupted white matter integrity have also been found in the brains of those who used cannabis regularly in adolescence. The risk of these negative outcomes is significantly lower if they start using cannabis later in life. Adolescence appears to be a window of vulnerability in which cannabis use can have particularly harmful effects.

Childhood Adversity: There is concerning evidence that childhood adversity, including poverty, trauma, abuse, neglect, and maltreatment, can disrupt brain development. Exposure to childhood adversity changes the structure of the brain, leading to altered connectivity between brain regions and reduced volumes of the hippocampus, prefrontal cortex, amygdala, corpus callosum, and other structures.[48] Like the other examples I've mentioned, the same outcomes are not seen when trauma or neglect is experienced in adulthood.[49] The specific age of exposure to adversity influences which structures are affected in the brain. For example, females exposed to physical or sexual abuse from ages nine to ten had a smaller corpus callosum, while those exposed between ages eleven to thirteen had smaller hippocampal volume.[50] I will talk about early childhood adversity and sport-related brain trauma in chapter 13.

HOW THIS RELATES TO REPETITIVE BRAIN TRAUMA IN YOUTH CONTACT SPORTS

Brain development is a complex dance involving multiple processes occurring at different rates and times over more than two decades. Whether good or bad, the choices, opportunities, trauma, or other events we experience during this time can permanently alter how our neurons and synapses develop and, ultimately, the form and function of our adult brain.[51]

The idea of disrupted development is not new. I gave several examples above, and countless others exist. It has been hypothesized that childhood may be a window of vulnerability during which concussions and repetitive brain trauma could significantly alter normal brain development, and I will discuss this in more detail in chapter 7. The many brain development processes happening, particularly between ages eight and twelve, may make it harder for the young brain to recover from injury.[52]

Though we still have a lot to learn, there is ample corroborating evidence to support the hypothesis that concussions and repetitive brain trauma can disrupt the brain development process. Disrupted development can occur throughout the body and in the brain from multiple causes. Even emotional trauma can alter development. Why would we think repetitive physical trauma to the brain would be any different?

Chapter Six

Why It's Not
All about Concussions

There must be a reduction in the number of head impacts. The continued focus on concussion and symptomatic recovery does not address the fundamental danger these activities pose to human health.
—Ann McKee, MD, chief of neuropathology, Boston VA Healthcare System; neuropathology core director, CTE Center, Boston University School of Medicine[1]

Much of the attention around brain safety in youth sports has focused on concussions. Concussions are often categorized as a "mild" brain injury because they don't immediately result in what we think of as life-threatening or even severe symptoms, like a coma, and the symptoms usually resolve within a few weeks. But a concussion is a serious injury to the brain that can significantly disrupt normal life and have lasting symptoms. Hiding or mistreating these injuries can result in life-altering consequences or even, in rare cases, death. Concussions need to be taken seriously, and the wealth of attention given to them in recent years is absolutely warranted.

Yet concussions are just *part* of the story of brain trauma in sports. The focus on these injuries has overshadowed the consequences of the hundreds of impacts incurred in a season and thousands sustained over a career of contact sports. Since the late 2000s, growing research has shown that repetitive impacts that occur with every tackle, block, header, check, or collision are not without consequence, even though they don't result in immediate symptoms. Changes have been seen in the brains of youth athletes, even over the course of one short season.

This chapter will start with an overview of concussions, debunking myths and highlighting key points all athletes, families, and coaches should know. Then I will shift the focus to what we know about the consequences of repetitive brain trauma and what it means for youth athletes.

CONCUSSIONS IN YOUTH SPORTS

A concussion is a type of traumatic brain injury resulting from a blow to the head or a blow to the body that causes the head to move rapidly, like a whiplash effect.[2] The brain is jostled and hits against prominent features within the skull. Axons connecting different parts of the brain are twisted and stretched, damaging neurons and leading to a cascade of chemical changes that disrupt normal transmission of signals in the brain.[3]

These concussive impacts can result in a variety of symptoms, such as blurred or double vision, headache, confusion, dizziness, balance issues, nausea, memory issues, sensitivity to light or noise, and difficulty concentrating.[4] Getting your bell rung, having a ding, or seeing stars were thought to be a normal part of some sports for decades, but now most medical professionals and scientists consider these to be concussions as well. Fatigue, difficulty sleeping, anxiety, and difficulty controlling emotions are often-overlooked symptoms in concussed youth athletes. Concussed athletes use more areas of the brain both at rest and when completing a task than those who don't have a concussion, in part due to damage to the white matter pathways in the brain.[5] White matter damage isn't visible on traditional brain imaging, but in research using special imaging techniques on concussed youth athletes, we can see damage in many brain pathways that can last for months after the injury.

Concussion Risk in Youth Sports

Concussion rates have risen across sports in recent years. Increased speed, roughness, and intensity of play even at young ages may be a factor, but it's also likely that improved education and understanding of the seriousness of these injuries is leading to more athletes reporting their concussion than ever before. Concussion rates in different sports vary, and sometimes by coincidence one group of athletes may simply have more or fewer injuries in a given year. When several studies conducted over time using similar methods are reviewed together, we can gain a better idea of both overall concussion rates and how different sports compare to each other.

In the United States, football is consistently the sport with the highest number and rate of concussions across all levels of play.[6] Around one in twenty youth players ages five to fourteen sustains a concussion each season,[7] and nearly 100,000 youth and 80,000 high school players suffer the injury each year.[8] Hockey most often has the highest rate after football, but youth hockey concussions have decreased over the last decade in the United States and Canada as a result of bans on checking before age thirteen.[9] For female athletes, soccer has the highest concussion rate at all levels of play.[10] Despite what some have claimed, nearly all studies have found that concussion rates in girls' and women's soccer are consistently lower than football. Lacrosse, wrestling, and competitive cheerleading also have concerning concussion rates. In lacrosse, the rates are significantly higher at the youth level than at the high school and college levels.[11] Rugby has concussion rates similar to football,[12] while youth Australian football has rates similar to those in hockey.[13]

In the same sport or sports with similar rules, female athletes are at a greater risk of sustaining a concussion compared to male athletes across all levels of play.[14] For example, despite experiencing fewer overall impacts at lower average accelerations, female hockey players tend to have similar concussion rates to their male counterparts.[15] Female soccer players are at around double the risk of sustaining a concussion compared to male players.[16] We don't know why females are at higher risk, but it may be due to better reporting by female athletes, weaker necks leading to higher accelerations, physiological differences, or a combination of factors.[17]

Most concussions happen as a result of player-to-player contact. Contact with tackling in football and rugby and with checking in hockey and lacrosse causes the majority of concussions.[18] In soccer, most concussions occur with head-to-head contact while attempting a header, followed by heading itself.[19] A higher overall number of concussions happen in practices than games simply because more time is spent in practices during the season. But in all sports, like the risk of sustaining a high-force impact, the concussion risk is higher in games.[20]

Common Misconceptions: Causes and Diagnosis of Concussions

"Concussions can only happen with high-force impacts." There is no known acceleration threshold above which the force of an impact is certain to cause a concussion or below which is certain to be safe. Impact force doesn't predict how bad the concussion symptoms will be either.[21] In college and high school athletes, accelerations above around 4000 rad/s^2 rotational and 102.5 g linear are likely to cause a concussion, but many brain injuries occur with forces much lower than that.[22] For example, a player may incur a hit of 80 g early in practice without symptoms and then sustain a hit later in practice at 40 g that results in a concussion. Certain athletes may be prone to these brain injuries at lower thresholds. Nine- to fourteen-year-old football players in one study sustained concussions with impacts at an average of 62.4 g linear and 2600 rad/s^2 rotational acceleration, much lower than the predicted high-risk accelerations in older players.[23] This suggests the developing brain of youth athletes may be at higher risk of sustaining a concussion with lower forces.

"It's not a concussion if you don't lose consciousness." It is a common misconception that you have to be knocked out, or lose consciousness, to have a concussion. That is not true, and, in fact, only about 10 percent of concussions actually result in a loss of consciousness.[24]

"All kids with concussions should have a brain scan." Brain CT scans and MRIs look completely normal with the vast majority of concussions, so these imaging techniques are not helpful for diagnosing the injury. Doctors should only recommend imaging if they suspect the patient may have a brain bleed due to vomiting, prolonged loss of consciousness, severe headache, or worsening symptoms.[25] The potential consequences of radiation exposure greatly outweigh the low likelihood of benefits of imaging for concussions. Advanced imaging methods are being developed in concussion research, but they aren't ready for the clinical setting.

"Blood tests can diagnose a concussion." Scientists are studying potential markers to diagnose a concussion with a simple blood test, but none exist yet. The only approved test is for emergency room use in adults with a more severe injury to determine if they need a CT scan.[26]

Concussion Management and Recovery

If an athlete is suspected of having a concussion, they should be immediately removed from the game or practice and evaluated by a medical professional with training in concussion diagnosis and management. Athletes who leave the game or practice immediately tend to return to their sport faster than those who keep playing, and continuing to play with a concussion raises the likelihood of having a prolonged recovery of over a month or more.[27] Those who continue to play after suffering a concussion are also more likely to have a higher number of symptoms and more severe symptoms compared to those who stopped playing immediately after their injury.

In the first twenty-four to forty-eight hours after sustaining a concussion, rest is best. After that, return to everyday life should be gradual.[28] Academic accommodations help student-athletes manage school while their brain recovers, and full return to school should always happen before return to sports. Once symptoms have resolved, a gradual return to play should be guided by a trained medical professional, progressing from limited light activity to sport-specific, non-contact play, to full-contact practice and games. If symptoms return at any point, the athlete should return to the previous step until they can complete that step without symptoms.

Nearly half of athletes are symptom-free within two weeks of the injury, and three-quarters have recovered by one month.[29] This is longer than we once thought. Compared to college athletes who played their sport in 1999 to 2001, athletes who played in 2014 to 2017 were held out about ten days longer.[30] This is actually a *good* thing. Returning to play too soon can increase the risk of sustaining a second concussion that often has more symptoms and a longer recovery.[31] In the earlier study, the second concussion usually happened within a week of the first. Forty-one percent fewer athletes in 2014 to 2017 suffered a second brain injury, and the delayed return was likely a key factor. Athletes who return while still having symptoms may perform worse in their sport due to delayed reaction time, impaired coordination, and other lingering deficits.[32] Of course, every athlete wants to get back into the game as soon as possible, but conservative management of these injuries is critically important to safe recovery, improved sport performance upon return, and prevention of future concussions.

Several factors can influence recovery time after a concussion. The rapidly developing brains of children and adolescents tend to take longer to recover than the adult brain.[33] Athletes with a previous concussion, especially multiple concussions, are also more likely to have a delayed recovery.[34] Female athletes also tend to have a greater number of and more severe symptoms and take longer to recover than male athletes.[35]

Even after all noticeable symptoms resolve and an athlete returns to play, the chemical changes and impaired signal transmission that occur with concussions can linger.[36] Changes in white matter, brain connectivity, and blood flow can persist a year or more after the injury.[37] Our brain does a great job of working around damage to accomplish a task, but that capacity is limited. For example, an athlete might seem fine with simple tasks, but deficits show with more complex tasks, like the physical demands of sports combined with game-related decision making.[38] This is likely a key reason why athletes are at greater risk of sustaining a lower extremity injury in the months or even years after a concussion.[39]

Common Misconceptions: Concussion Recovery and Return to Play

"A player can safely return to play if their concussion symptoms last less than fifteen minutes." This used to be common practice, but we now know that athletes should never return to play on the day of the injury. Youth athletes are far more likely than high school athletes to return to play less than twenty-four hours after a concussion,[40] likely due in large part to a lack of trained medical personnel at youth events. Returning to play before symptoms resolve can have dire consequences. Though rare, second impact syndrome can occur if a young athlete sustains a second brain injury before they fully recover from the first.[41] It is thought that the second impact ultimately causes unregulated blood flow and swelling in the brain that is fatal in around half of cases.

"You should wake a concussed person up throughout the first night to make sure they're okay." This also used to be common practice, but it is no longer recommended. Sleep is critical for recovery in athletes of all ages, and a lack of sleep after a concussion can actually increase the severity of symptoms.[42] If a concussed athlete is unusually drowsy or unable to stay awake, it may be cause for concern, and you should call a doctor.

"Concussed athletes should stay in a dark room with little mental or physical stimulation." Mild stimulation can actually be helpful following a concussion. The key is to avoid things that make the symptoms worse, which could include using computers and other devices or physical or mental overexertion. Growing research shows prolonged complete rest can actually increase symptoms and lengthen recovery from a concussion, while short bouts of very light exercise may actually help with recovery. [43] However, this must be done the right way with the right progression under the guidance of a qualified medical professional.

"Passing a computerized test means an athlete is ready to play." Athletes and parents will often ask for a computerized neurocognitive test, like the ImPACT, thinking that, if they pass, they must be ready to return to play. But it doesn't work that way. These tests often have lower reliability in young athletes than adults, so clinicians need to ensure they are using age-appropriate tests. [44] Even if the athlete has a baseline test to compare to postconcussion performance, it may not be valid. Some athletes intentionally perform poorly on the baseline so they don't have to score as high during recovery to reach preinjury levels. [45] As a result, they may be allowed to return to play sooner than they should. While a computerized test can give useful information about the patient's recovery, a good clinician will never rely solely on it, or any one test, to make a return to play decision. Instead, they will consider the entire clinical exam when making that decision.

Special Considerations for Concussions in Children and Adolescents

In sports, children and adolescents tend to be at higher risk of getting a concussion, taking longer to recover from the injury, and having poorer outcomes compared to adults. [46] As discussed in the previous chapter, concussions in children and teens may disrupt the typical trajectory of brain development, potentially resulting in often subtle lasting consequences. [47] Even if a concussed child has a full recovery and returns to preinjury levels, they may have fallen behind their peers who continued maturing over that time. Better concussion management can help youth athletes make a quicker and safer return to normal activity. Concussion management should be age appropriate and conservative in young athletes. An eight-year-old's brain is different than that of a twelve-year-old or an eighteen-year-old.

CONSEQUENCES OF REPETITIVE SUBCONCUSSIVE BRAIN TRAUMA

It was long thought that the routine head impacts inherent to many contact sports were harmless if they didn't result in immediate symptoms. We now know these repetitive impacts can have both immediate and lasting consequences for the brain. They are often referred to as subconcussive impacts because they don't result in concussion symptoms. It isn't the best term to describe these hits, given that there are no known lower thresholds of force for sustaining a concussion. Even so, it is a common descriptive term, and I will use it throughout this book.

Short-Term Exposure to Repetitive Subconcussive Impacts

Repetitive subconcussive impacts can change the brain over the course of just one season even if the athlete did not have a concussion. A variety of imaging methods and other tests have been used to study the effects of these impacts. The studies typically perform baseline tests on each athlete before the season begins and then compare them to tests after the season has ended.

Diffusion tensor imaging, or DTI, is a type of MRI that gives information about the white matter pathways in the brain. At the high school and college level, a growing number of DTI studies have shown evidence of damage to white matter pathways after one season of play in several sports, including football, hockey, and soccer.[48] In one study of college football players, the markers suggestive of white matter damage did not return to preseason levels even six months after the season.[49] White matter changes are also evident in the brains of eight- to thirteen-year-old football players after one short season of youth football.[50]

Functional MRI, or fMRI, can be used to examine underlying physiology, connectivity, and blood flow in brain networks. Using this method, alterations in connectivity have been found in youth, high school, and college football players after one season.[51] Researchers at the University of Texas Southwestern Medical Center reported that a single season of youth and high school football may disrupt the synaptic pruning process.[52] This can lead to larger overall volumes and inefficient connectivity in the prefrontal region of the brain. Changes in blood flow have been detected using fMRI in the brains of female high school soccer players after one season, and the altered blood flow lingered until around five months after the season ended.[53]

Many other studies have shown changes in the brain after a single season of repetitive impacts. For example, changes in gray matter volumes have been shown to persist at least one month after a college football season.[54] Altered levels of substances in the blood and chemical levels in the brain have been reported in high school and college football players, suggesting that a season of repetitive impacts can damage neurons in the brain.[55] Repetitive subconcussive trauma may also disrupt the blood-brain barrier, which protects the brain by only allowing certain substances to leave blood vessels and enter the space around the neurons.[56] Blood-brain barrier disruption may have implications for the development of CTE, but more on that in chapter 8.

Repetitive impacts can also affect the brain over short time spans. Male and female college rugby players can have connectivity changes on fMRI after a single match,[57] while disruptions in connectivity, physiology, and motor control have been observed after routine soccer heading.[58]

Despite physical changes observed in the brains of athletes after repetitive subconcussive impacts, functional deficits and symptoms from these impacts are less clear. Differences in reaction time, processing speed, memory, balance, impulse control, and attention have been observed in contact sport athletes at the high school and college level after one or two seasons.[59] Yet many studies have found no deficits or even improvement in various functions after exposure to a season of repetitive subconcussive impacts.[60]

How can there be clear visible changes in the brain but no measurable changes in brain function? There are a few potential explanations. First, the tests used in the studies may not be capable of identifying subtle deficits from subconcussive impacts, but they may be observed with more complex tasks. It's also possible that there are simply no deficits to observe. The brain may be able to compensate for slight alterations resulting from these impacts, raising the question of how concerning the changes observed in the brain really are. However, short-term compensation may also hide initial symptoms and deficits that won't become evident until later in life, as normal aging or neurodegenerative disease takes its toll. Right now, we just don't know.

Expected improvement may also mask deficits from repetitive subconcussive trauma. Children and adolescents are supposed to be improving in their cognition and behavioral control due to typical development, and some improvements arise with greater athleticism from training. Not seeing a decline in performance doesn't mean that deficits aren't there. Research supports this. Multiple studies have shown less improvement in contact sport athletes preseason to postseason in several cognitive functions compared to non–contact sport athletes.[61] A lack of typical improvement may be a sign that brain function is affected, and staying the same or improving less than other kids who didn't sustain repetitive brain trauma could actually be a sign of slowed or impaired development.

The total number of impacts a person sustains influences the changes observed in the brain as well as functional deficits and other symptoms. Greater alterations in blood flow, metabolism, and chemical levels in the brain as well as more evidence of white matter damage have been found in soccer and football players with the most exposure to repetitive impacts in the previous year or season.[62] Poorer reaction time, memory, and attention were related to a higher number of headers performed by soccer players over time as well.[63] Not surprisingly, a higher number of impacts seems to be worse for the brain.

Repetitive Subconcussive Impacts over Years of Play

Repetitive subconcussive impacts accumulated over a career cause lasting damage to the brain. Some of these consequences are visible while the athlete is still playing their sport, and others have been observed in former athletes years after their retirement. My colleagues and I at the Boston University (BU) CTE Center and the Psychiatry Neuroimaging Laboratory at Harvard Medical School observed poor executive functions in former college and NFL players as well as smaller volumes of the hippocampus and amygdala in NFL players.[64] White matter damage, altered functional connectivity, thinning of the cortex, poorer cognitive performance, and depression have also been observed in professional soccer, rugby, and football players.[65]

We don't know if a certain number of impacts leads to later-life functional deficits or brain degeneration. Dr. Philip Montenigro and colleagues at the BU CTE Center used reported playing history and position along with data from accelerometer studies to estimate the number of impacts sustained by former high school and college football players over their football career.[66] The average player sustained an estimated 5,806 impacts. When players reached a threshold between 1,800 and 2,400 estimated impacts, their risk of having difficulties with executive functions, regulating behavior, depression, and apathy nearly doubled. To be clear, incurring a number of impacts below the threshold wasn't necessarily safe, but the risk increased significantly after reaching that threshold. Above the threshold, the risk doubled again with an additional 2,800 hits. The more subconcussive impacts sustained over a career, the greater the risk of lasting consequences.

Evidence of cumulative damage from years of repetitive impacts can even be seen in active high school athletes. Researchers observed that athletes who played high-contact sports had slower processing speed and reaction time, worse impulse control, and in some cases, memory issues when compared to low-contact sport athletes even before the season started.[67] Football linemen, the position that tends to experience the most impacts over the course of a season, had greater difficulty with all of those functions than players at other positions.[68] The repetitive impacts sustained over years of play may start to take a toll even in young athletes.

Other research has found no negative consequences of repetitive impacts in high school sports. Unfortunately, some have used these findings to argue contact sports are safe for the brain, but these studies should be interpreted with caution. Two studies examined men who were in seventh through twelfth grade during the 1994 to 1995 school year.[69] Their *intention* to play football, hockey, wrestling, or soccer that year was not related to cognition or depression almost fifteen years later. However, researchers didn't verify if the men actually played the sport, and there was no information about the total number of years they played or the age they started playing the sport. These factors limit how meaningful the results might be for current or future high school athletes.

In another study, high school football players in Wisconsin who graduated in 1957 did not have an increased risk of depression or cognitive issues compared to nonathletes or non–contact sport athletes.[70] The game has changed quite a bit since that time. Many of the athletes only played for one year in high school, and the study did not indicate whether they played football before high school, though fewer youth leagues existed at the time. The findings really suggest that playing a few years of high school football in the 1950s was not likely to lead to later-life cognitive difficulties and depression. This is a good thing, and it fits with the idea that experiencing fewer impacts means an athlete is at lower risk of having later-life difficulties. Yet the study

says little about playing high school football today, especially combined with several years of youth play prior to high school.

HOW SUBCONCUSSIVE IMPACTS MAY INCREASE
CONCUSSION RISK

There is growing evidence that the subconcussive impacts sustained in
the time leading up to a concussion may play a key role in causing the
concussion. For example, college football and women's hockey players
who sustained a concussion had experienced significantly more impacts on the day they were injured compared to those who were not
injured.[71] Concussed athletes have also been shown to sustain more
impacts in the week or season leading up to the injury compared to
athletes who were not injured.[72]

Timing between individual subconcussive impacts may be another
factor increasing concussion risk.[73] It takes time for the brain to return
to normal balance after trauma. The more damage an impact causes, the
longer it will take for that balance to be restored. If the brain isn't given
enough time to recover before another hit occurs, the second impact
could impede recovery from the first, and so on as hits continue. It
might not lead to a concussion right away, but as more hits occur before
full recovery is reached, it may eventually take less force with a later
impact to get a concussion.

CONCERN ABOUT REPETITIVE SUBCONCUSSIVE IMPACTS
IN YOUTH SPORTS

Concussions are serious injuries, and it is critical that they are diagnosed and managed appropriately. However, the repetitive impacts that
transmit forces to the brain with every hit, and nearly every play in
some sports, can also cause lasting damage to the brain. We tend to
focus on the immediate consequences of injuries in sport, but we often
don't think about consequences years down the road. And if there are
no obvious signs of injury right after the impact, no damage is done,
right? Wrong. We need to be just as concerned about repetitive subconcussive impacts in youth sports as we are about concussions. In the next
chapter you will learn that, at the youth level, we have to worry about
the consequences these impacts may have on brain development. And
in chapter 8, you will see that starting at a younger age means more

accumulated impacts over their careers, increasing the risk for developing CTE. Simply waiting until adolescence to start playing the full-contact version of a sport, along with substantially reducing impacts in practice, can go a long way toward minimizing negative consequences of repetitive subconcussive impacts.

Chapter Seven

Why Head Impacts in Youth Sports May Be Disrupting Brain Development

The body, the brain, the skull is not developed in your teens and single digits. I cringe. I see these little kids get tackled, and the helmet is bigger than everything else on the kid combined. They look like they're going to break in half.
—Brett Favre, NFL Hall of Fame quarterback [1]

Every fall over two million youth boys (and a growing number of girls) put on football pads and helmets and hit the gridiron. [2] Parents and grandparents cheer them on as they try to imitate the stars they watch play on television. But, behind the cheers, some parents worry about the brain trauma their child may sustain playing the sport.

At this point in the book you have learned that incurring repetitive head impacts, whether over a season or a career, can create lasting changes in brain anatomy and function. You have learned that young boys and girls can incur hundreds of these hits in just one season of youth sports. You have also learned that the young brain is particularly vulnerable. What happens when all of these factors happen at once, when kids are hitting their heads repeatedly in youth contact sports at a time when their brain is rapidly developing?

I became interested in studying brain trauma in sports during my time working with young athletes, and I wanted to understand how these repetitive impacts might uniquely affect a brain that is rapidly maturing. Studies had looked at concussions in youth athletes, but until I teamed up with my colleague Dr. Alex Bourlas and others at the CTE Center, no one had investigated the long-term consequences of repetitive subconcussive impacts in youth. We published our first study on this topic in 2015, and several have followed since then.

The findings of these studies have significant implications for young athletes playing contact sports. That's why it is critical that the studies are designed the right way. You could use a thousand different tests in an analysis, but if you aren't using the *right* tests with the *right* methods, the findings may be meaningless. For example, if you want to test a person's ability to do calculus, you don't give them a simple addition or subtraction problem. You give them a calculus problem. When it comes to concussive and subconcussive brain trauma in youth sports, studies must be designed based on what we know about typical brain development trajectories.

In this chapter I will explain what we have learned in our research on repetitive impacts to the developing brain. I will also discuss studies on younger athletes with differing findings and explain the picture that may be forming when all of this research is considered together.

LONG-TERM CONSEQUENCES OF REPETITIVE SUBCONCUSSIVE IMPACTS TO THE DEVELOPING BRAIN

My colleagues and I conducted three studies of the long-term consequences of repetitive impacts in youth football in a group of former NFL football players between the ages of forty and sixty-five. While these players were older at the time of the research, we examined their current function and brain structure with respect to their age when they started playing tackle football. That allowed us to investigate potential later-life consequences of the impacts they experienced when they were young. The former NFL players who started playing at a younger age usually played more years of football. We know that more years of play likely means more career impacts, which increases the likelihood of having a variety of symptoms later in life.[3] We had to account for this in our research to ensure any differences we found between groups were due to age they started playing tackle football and not the number of years they played. We also accounted for the player's age or decade they played in, as football has changed a lot over time.

First, we examined whether or not the age that the former NFL players started playing influenced how well their brain was working to reason, inhibit impulses, problem solve, learn, and more.[4] As I mentioned in chapter 5, there is a lot happening in a boy's brain between ages eight and twelve, with many important structures and processes reaching a peak during that time. Because of this, we divided the former NFL players into two groups: those who started playing tackle football before age twelve and those who started playing at age twelve or later. The former NFL players who began playing football before age twelve had significantly more trouble with executive functions, greater difficulties learning and remembering a list of words, and scored lower on a measure of estimated IQ than those who waited until they were older to begin playing the game. This study provided the first evidence that repetitive hits to the head through youth football can have lasting consequences.

Next, we wanted to know if repetitive impacts at a young age caused lasting physical changes to the brain.[5] We started by studying the corpus callosum, the white matter pathway sending information between the left and right hemispheres of the brain. As I mentioned in chapter 5, this pathway is particularly vulnerable to brain trauma, and it undergoes a critical period of rapid development between ages eight and twelve, especially in the regions of the pathway closest to the front of the brain. Fitting with this developmental milestone, we found evidence of potential damage to axons in parts of the corpus callosum near the front of the brain in former NFL players who started playing before age twelve. Some of this evidence suggested that those who started tackling at a younger age may have had less myelin on their axons. It's possible that repetitive subconcussive impacts from youth tackle football may have disrupted the myelination process, resulting in a permanently thinner layer of myelin than nature had intended. We also found that the portion of the corpus callosum near the front of the brain showed worse damage the older the former player was, but this was greater in the group that began playing before age twelve. Disrupted myelination or other effects from repetitive impacts in childhood may leave the pathway more vulnerable to the effects of aging or degeneration later in life.

Next, we measured the size of the thalamus in the former NFL players.[6] The thalamus is a structure deep in the brain that serves as an important relay station. It receives information from one part of the brain, processes it, and sends the information to other parts of the brain.

The thalamus increases in volume into the late teen years.[7] It doesn't have a developmental peak around age twelve, so it didn't make sense to use that cutoff in this study. Instead, we simply looked for an association between the age they started playing and the size of their thalamus. We found that the younger the person was when they began playing tackle football, the smaller their right thalamus was. In addition, the more years of football a former NFL athlete played, the smaller their thalamus was. More years played likely means the individual experienced more hits to the head, and consistent with other research, it seems that a greater number of hits is associated with reduced size of this important structure. Notably, the effect of the age they started playing was nearly *double* the effect of the number of years they played, meaning the age they started had a bigger influence on their thalamus size.

Like all research, these studies have limitations, including the fact that all of these former NFL players were at high risk for having CTE based on their symptoms and their long football careers. Damage already present potentially due to CTE, or simply from years of repetitive impacts, could have made it impossible to detect subtle damage from playing football at a young age. But that wasn't the case. Instead, we saw deficits in those who started playing at a younger age *despite* the fact that they were at high risk for having CTE.

It's important to remember that these types of studies must be designed based on what we know about typical peaks and timing in brain development. Another research group studied former NFL players and found no relationship between the number of years of football they played before high school and negative later-life consequences.[8] However, they used measures I wouldn't expect to differ by the age of first exposure to repetitive impacts. For example, they used a measure that combined all white matter of the brain together, despite the fact that some pathways peak in childhood and others continue developing past age thirty. This likely washed out any potential findings they could have seen had they focused on a specific pathway and designed the study based on its developmental path. Another structure they studied reaches its adult form by six months old, so there is no reason to expect differences in that structure based on the age the impacts began. We can't expect a significant finding with every measure, and no study is perfect. Yet it is critical that any study examining the consequences of repetitive impacts in children be designed based on what we know about typical brain development.

All of the above studies only included former NFL football players. We couldn't say whether the findings applied to athletes who only play through the youth or high school levels. To address this limitation, we expanded our next study to include amateur players as well. Of the 214 former tackle football players we studied, around half played through college, and 20 percent only played through high school.[9] We found that former tackle football players who started playing before age twelve reported more symptoms of depression and apathy and greater difficulties with executive functions than those who began playing at an older age. Cognition did not differ between groups, perhaps because the measure isn't sensitive enough to detect subtle changes from exposure to repetitive head impacts or because there were simply no differences to find. Nevertheless, those who began playing before age twelve were at two times greater odds of reporting clinically impaired executive functioning and three times greater odds of reporting clinically meaningful depressive symptoms. That means the former players met a level of impairment that would be concerning to a doctor.

We also looked at the whole group without the age cutoff and found that the younger they started playing football, the worse they scored on the measures of depressive symptoms, apathy symptoms, and behavioral aspects of executive function, like impulsivity and inhibition. But when using the age twelve cutoff, the results were stronger than when we looked at the specific age they started playing. This lines up with what we know about critical periods of brain development. For example, the amygdala reaches a peak volume around age twelve, and this structure is thought to be involved in depression and apathy.

Notably, the findings held true regardless of the number of years played or the level of play reached. The difficulties associated with incurring repetitive impacts while playing football at a young age were the same whether the athletes reached the high school, college, or professional level.

A few other studies have investigated potential consequences of exposure to repetitive subconcussive impacts through sports at a young age. Another study of former NFL players found no effect of age of first exposure on self-reported cognition-related quality of life, anxiety, or depression, though they only used a two-question initial screening tool for depression and anxiety, not a comprehensive assessment.[10] Active and retired professional boxers or mixed martial arts fighters have also been studied based on the age they started fighting.[11] Earlier exposure to fighting was related to smaller volumes of the hippocampus, corpus callosum, and, in some cases, the amygdala as well as worse processing speed, balance, impulsivity, and depression. Youth athletes can begin participating in organized combat sports training at a young age, but it is important to note that the authors did not provide ages that the athletes in the study began fighting. Though the study supports the idea that repetitive impacts at a younger age can have greater consequences, we should interpret the findings with caution.

Other studies have examined the consequences of repetitive impacts in childhood and found no consequences in active high school and college athletes on cognitive, mood, behavior, balance, or other measures.[12] It is very possible that repetitive impacts in youth had no negative effects in the groups examined in these studies. Yet there are a few important points to consider.

Several studies used the computerized test ImPACT, but that may not be a useful measure. While the computerized test is valid and often used with concussions,[13] we don't know if it is sensitive enough to detect subtle differences in brain function from repetitive subconcussive impacts. Practice effects from having taken the test several times can also play a role. Athletes in contact sports with a higher risk of concussions are more likely than non–contact sport athletes to have taken one or more baseline ImPACT tests in high school and, as a result, more likely to have improved from practice.[14] These are important factors to consider, and we need more research using thorough neuropsychological testing in current athletes with respect to the age they started playing contact sports.

As I said before, the design of these studies needs to be rooted in what we know about typical brain development. Different functions measured by ImPACT and other measures used in two studies follow different developmental trajectories, some of which don't have a critical period around age twelve. The researchers likely used the age twelve cutoff because that is what we used in our studies, which is a common and rational thing to do. But in this research, groupings should be based on the development of the specific structure or function being examined. Also, the average age of the subjects was between seventeen and nineteen years old, but the brain does not fully mature until the early to midtwenties. We may not be able to detect subtle differences due to youth exposure to repetitive subconcussive impacts in a function that isn't fully developed yet. Ultimately, more research rooted in neurodevelopment is needed so that we can understand how repetitive head impacts in youth sports may be affecting our children throughout their lives.

WHAT DOES THIS MEAN FOR KIDS WHO WANT TO PLAY CONTACT SPORTS?

Taking all of the research on repetitive subconcussive impacts in childhood together, an intriguing possibility is starting to emerge. We saw deficits in brain function and structure later in life in older individuals who started playing tackle football at a younger age. Yet studies of current high school and college contact sport athletes did not observe these deficits. Why would we see deficits from similar exposure in older former athletes and not in current teen and young adult athletes? It's possible that repetitive impacts in youth may affect our brain's reserve.

Imagine two identical cars driving down the highway. Both started the trip at the same place, but one started with a full tank of gas while the other started with the tank only half full. Both vehicles can travel normally for many miles, but the second car will run out of gas first and won't be able to travel as far. Now let's say that gas tank is like our brain. In childhood and adolescence, we are in the process of filling the tank, laying down myelin and trying to refine connections in the best possible way. Repetitive subconcussive impacts may disrupt this process, hindering our ability to put as much neuronal "fuel in the tank" as possible. It may be like we are starting our trip into adulthood without a full tank of gas. We can still function well for many years, but our brain is at a disadvantage with degenerative changes from either normal aging or disease. If we start with more neuronal fuel in our brain's tank, like myelin, synapses, and efficient connectivity, we can afford to lose more with degenerative changes before any symptoms begin to show. But if we have fewer connections to begin with, it takes less damage and pathology before we develop symptoms.

The idea that something could put our brain at a disadvantage and reduce our reserved neuronal "fuel" is not new. Alcohol dependence, HIV-related inflammation, chemotherapy, and other environmental factors can have an effect on the brain, and they have been associated with accelerated brain aging and earlier onset of disease symptoms.[15] Exposure to repetitive subconcussive brain trauma in childhood may be another factor that puts the brain at a disadvantage and accelerates the onset of symptoms from aging or disease.

Childhood is a time when the brain is rapidly developing. If we disrupt that process, we may reduce the brain's total reserve. It may not affect us through early or middle adulthood. However, as our reserve starts to decline with the normal aging process or disease, it takes less time before we reach a point where we have lost too much, and we start to have symptoms. This could explain why exposure to repetitive impacts in youth contact sports had no consequences in studies of younger athletes but related deficits were observed in older, retired athletes. A child who starts playing a contact sport today at age eight may not see the consequences of these head impacts for fifty years, but when they do arise, they can be devastating.

IN SUMMARY, DON'T HIT YOUR HEAD A LOT AS A KID

Some people don't want to believe that repetitive impacts in youth sports could affect us when we are older. I often hear the argument: "I played at a young age and I'm fine." I ask, are they fine? Yeah, they probably are. But isn't it *possible* that some traits passed off as personality flaws may actually be related to repetitive brain trauma in youth? Maybe a man's depression symptoms in his forties are related to repetitive impacts he took as a child in youth football, or a woman's subtle cognitive issues in her fifties could be related to years of impacts in youth rugby. Sure, there are many different causes of depression and cognitive issues, and we have much to learn on this topic. But we shouldn't ignore the possibility that repetitive subconcussive trauma in childhood could be a cause. We just don't tend to think about it because the repetitive impacts happened a long time ago as a normal part of a fun activity.

There is so much development and maturation happening in a child's brain, and it makes sense that repetitive impacts could disrupt these processes, resulting in lasting consequences. We will never eliminate every hit and every concussion. Kids are kids. They will fall, they will run into things, and they will hit their head every once in a while. But we can greatly reduce the hits they experience by taking away unnecessary exposure in contact sports. It would be concerning if a child hit their head against a wall 250 times over twelve weeks. So why is it okay in sports?

Yet this research is just in its infancy, and there is so much more that we need to learn. There may be factors that make one youth athlete more or less vulnerable to the effects of these impacts. Most work on this topic has been on football players. We need to study the effects of repetitive impacts in youth athletes that play other high-risk sports, especially females. While we need to continue working to discover the answers to these questions, we can take a collective look at the findings of these studies combined with the supporting data on disrupted development in the brain and other body systems and make a commonsense conclusion: repetitive hits to the head are not good for the developing brain.

I want to make one final point very clear: this research does *not* suggest that it is safe to sustain repetitive impacts after age twelve. Childhood might be one critical period in which repetitive subconcussive trauma could have greater consequences. But different brain structures develop at different rates, and structures that continue to develop into adolescence and adulthood can still be vulnerable to repetitive trauma. Experiencing subconcussive impacts at any age, including in adulthood, could lead to CTE or other consequences. In general, it just isn't a good idea to hit our heads over and over again. Our brain controls everything, from our ability to think and reason to our personality and mood to our ability to smile or walk. Having a healthy brain is an important component of living a healthy life. We should do everything we can to protect it.

Chapter Eight

Why CTE Is More Than an NFL Problem, and What It Means for Youth Sports

The only common factor we have that links boxers with American footballers with ice hockey with soccer with rugby with wrestling with domestic violence with circus performers is exposure to head injury and head impacts. So it's difficult to square that assumption that there is a lack of evidence to support this.
                    —Dr. Willie Stewart, neuropathologist, University of Glasgow [1]

Much of the concern around brain injury in sports centers on the neurodegenerative disease chronic traumatic encephalopathy, or CTE. CTE is a neurodegenerative disease that may be caused, in part, by repetitive brain trauma, whether concussive or subconcussive.[2] It was first described in boxers in 1928 by New Jersey pathologist Dr. Harrison Martland.[3] It was referred to as "punch drunk" or "dementia pugilistica," as it was originally diagnosed in boxers. The term *chronic traumatic encephalopathy* was first used in 1940.[4] In 1933 the NCAA admitted that football players could become "punch drunk."[5] Yet it wasn't until 2005 that CTE gained national attention, when Dr. Bennet Omalu published the first diagnosed case in a former NFL player, Mike Webster.[6]

There is a lot that could be said about CTE, and we still have a lot to learn. This chapter will provide an overview of what we know and don't know about the disease, with a focus on the risk for youth athletes. CTE is not only a disease of former professional athletes. It has been diagnosed in teenagers and athletes who only played a few years of their sport at the high school level. How concerned should we be about young athletes getting CTE from youth contact sports?

WHAT IS CTE?

CTE is what we call a tauopathy, which means a protein called tau plays a key role in the disease process.[7] Tau is an important part of the healthy brain. Its job is to stabilize and support the part of the neuron responsible for carrying substances through the axon from one part of the brain to another.[8] In CTE, and in other tauopathies like Alzheimer's disease, the tau becomes tangled, clumped together, and essentially toxic, ultimately resulting in death of the neuron.

If you were to look at the whole brain of an individual with advanced CTE and compare it to a typical, healthy brain of someone the same age, you would notice signs that neurons have died, including enlarged spaces in the brain and a decreased overall size of the brain.[9] Structures in the brain that are affected by the disease, such as the hippocampus and amygdala, decrease in size, too, and loss of neurons may also be noticeable in the brainstem. However, in early, less advanced cases, the brain may appear relatively normal to the eye.

Most changes in the brain from CTE can only be seen with a microscope. Dr. Ann McKee is the chief or neuropathology for the Boston VA Healthcare System and director of the Neuropathology Core at the BU CTE Center. Dr. McKee has examined more brains of individuals with CTE than anyone in the world, and she developed a four-stage system for describing the severity of the disease.[10] In Stage I, the earliest stage, the tau is found in specific regions of the frontal lobes. It tends to surround blood vessels at the deepest parts of the grooves, or sulci, in the prefrontal cortex. Damage to axons can be seen in even the earliest cases of CTE, including a loss of myelin. In Stage II, tau is widespread in regions of the frontal lobe, and by Stage III it has infiltrated hippocampus and amygdala in the temporal lobe, near the ears. Other structures deep in the brain and areas of the brainstem are also increasingly affected with disease progression. In Stage IV, most of, if not the entire brain is teeming with toxic tau tangles.

The development and distribution of the tau tangles may be related to the stresses on the brain that occur with impacts. Impact forces cause a great amount of strain at the deepest part of the sulci on the surface of the brain.[11] These physical stresses might explain why the tau first accumulates in that location in CTE. Places where different types of tissue meet also feel high strain with impact forces, such as where the brain tissue meets the tissue that makes up blood vessels. As I mentioned in chapter 6, repetitive brain trauma can disrupt the blood-brain barrier. Though not proven yet, evidence suggests that damage to the blood-brain barrier may be involved in the processes leading to the development of CTE.[12]

Several other neurodegenerative diseases are tauopathies, including Alzheimer's disease, and many of the changes in the brain I described for CTE occur in other diseases too. Despite these similarities, CTE is its own distinct disease.[13] It differs from Alzheimer's disease in many ways.[14] For example, the tau protein in Alzheimer's disease doesn't surround small blood vessels as it does in CTE. Alzheimer's disease also progresses differently, affecting parts of the brain in a different order than CTE. Another key difference is the presence of an additional protein called beta amyloid. While this protein is found in some CTE cases, it tends to be a different form of the protein and in older individuals. A person can also have both CTE and Alzheimer's disease or another neurodegenerative disease at the same time.

The earliest stage of CTE is usually asymptomatic, meaning the disease is present in the brain, but the individual doesn't have any symptoms.[15] In most neurodegenerative conditions, the loss of neurons in the brain starts years before symptoms arise.[16] CTE is likely no exception. This is one reason we need to find a way to diagnose the disease during life. If we know someone might be at high risk and we can see the tau in their brain before they start having symptoms, we could potentially treat the disease early (if a treatment existed) and prevent it from ever progressing to the point of developing symptoms.

When symptoms do arise, which usually occurs in middle age, they fall in the categories of behavior, mood, or cognitive function.[17] Memory issues and difficulties with executive function, attention, and concentration are common cognitive symptoms. A lack of inhibition and impulse control, having a short fuse, verbal or physical violence, and aggression are common behavioral symptoms. Mood-related symptoms include depression, irritability, anxiety, and suicidality. Some patients also have motor symptoms that are similar to Parkinson's disease, including difficulty with balance and slowed gait, while others have a variant similar to amyotrophic lateral sclerosis, also known as ALS or Lou Gehrig's disease. Headaches are common, even in early stages of

CTE. In some cases, it's difficult to know if symptoms like headaches were actually from the disease or if they were lingering from a previous concussion or recent exposure to repetitive head impacts.

Current or former athletes struggling with issues like headaches, depression, or anxiety should *not* assume that these are symptoms of CTE. In fact, they are probably more likely to be lingering symptoms of a previous concussion or simply the result of other causes. Anxiety and depression are common, and headaches can have many origins. Regardless of the cause of these symptoms, existing treatments can help. Although there are no treatments for CTE at this time, there are successful treatments for depression, anxiety, and other symptoms.

DIAGNOSING CTE

Despite what you may have heard in the news, at this time CTE can only be diagnosed by examining the brain after death.[18] Not being able to diagnose the disease during life makes it difficult if not impossible to study certain aspects of the disease, like prevalence and risk factors. Most of what we know about CTE symptoms has come from interviews with loved ones of people who were diagnosed after death. No treatments exist at this time, but researchers can't test a potential treatment if they don't know for sure who has the disease.

Scientists are making progress toward diagnosing CTE in the living. Early studies have found higher tau levels in the blood and cerebrospinal fluid, the fluid that surrounds the brain and spinal cord, in former NFL players with CTE-like symptoms.[19] Tau could also be in the blood or cerebrospinal fluid in other tauopathies, but these relatively inexpensive tests along with the patient's history and clinical examination could be used to diagnose CTE in the future.

A new imaging method also has great potential.[20] First, the patient receives an injection of a radioactive material, called a ligand, that binds to the tau protein in the brain. Then they undergo a positron emission tomography, or PET, scan. The radioactive ligand causes the tau in the brain to light up on the scan. Radioactive ligands also exist that bind to beta amyloid, the other protein in Alzheimer's disease. If a patient with CTE symptoms received one scan that showed the presence of tau and another scan that showed no amyloid, it would strongly suggest a diagnosis of CTE. This would be the gold standard for diagnosing CTE in the living.

It is important to be cautious with claims of an ability to diagnose CTE using these scans now. In 2013 several former NFL players said they were diagnosed with CTE based on a PET scan they had at UCLA.[21] However, this small study used a ligand that binds not only to tau but also to beta amyloid, making it difficult to determine if the athlete had CTE or Alzheimer's disease. It also included just five living former players. Researchers are investigating other ligands that bind only to tau. An early PET study found evidence of tau being visible in the brains of living former NFL players, with the amount of tau in the brain being correlated with the total number of years they played football.[22] Yet, no matter what ligand is used, a large number of these scans have to be compared with the findings of an examination of the player's brain after death before we can know for sure that the scan is right. It will still be quite a while before these scans will be proven to diagnose CTE and be available clinically.

WE DON'T KNOW HOW COMMON CTE IS

The prevalence of CTE has been widely distorted in the media on both extremes, with some claiming it's extremely rare and others claiming nearly every football player has it. At this time, all verified cases of CTE come from brain banks, where generous donors or families have chosen to donate their or their loved one's brain for examination after their death. The brains can be examined at the group level to study features of the disease. However, we can't learn actual prevalence from these studies because the sample is very biased toward a greater likelihood of finding CTE. Would you think to donate the brain of your loved one if they lived a healthy life and died of natural causes? Probably not. Most brain donations occur out of concern that the person had CTE, so it makes sense that the brain bank would find a high prevalence of CTE in their sample. That does not make the sample representative of all contact sport athletes.

From what we know now, neither of the extremes are true. In 2017, a team led by Dr. McKee diagnosed CTE in 110 out of 111 former NFL players whose brains were donated to the Veterans Affairs–BU–Concussion Legacy Foundation brain bank.[23] This is striking, but despite how the media portrayed it, this *does not* mean nearly all NFL players will get CTE. The goal of the study, which the authors clearly explained, was to describe what CTE looks like in the brains of football players, not to give any information on prevalence of the disease.

However, we can use that number to calculate an estimated prevalence. If only the 110 diagnosed players had the disease out of all NFL players who died in the same years as the brain donors, the prevalence of the disease would be nearly 10 percent.[24] This is quite high for a neurodegenerative disease.[25] Another estimate using approximate numbers of total players over the last fifty years of NFL football (not just those who died), suggests a minimum of four to thirteen CTE cases per one thousand NFL players. The Occupational Safety and Health Administration regulates occupations with a risk of one in one thousand or higher.[26] It is extremely unlikely that only the 110 players whose brains happened to be examined had the disease and all others who played over that time did not, suggesting these numbers likely underestimate the actual prevalence in the NFL population. Still, we are not able to make any meaningful estimates at this time regarding those who played amateur football or those who played other sports.

Given that we cannot diagnose CTE in the living, it's likely that some people who were diagnosed with Alzheimer's disease, Parkinson's disease, or other diseases during life actually had CTE. Former NFL players and professional soccer players are three times more likely to die of neurodegenerative causes than the general population and at least four times more likely to die of ALS, despite the fact that these athletes have a lower risk of dying from other causes.[27]

WHO IS AT RISK FOR GETTING CTE?

Most people have heard of CTE in the media, with high-profile deaths of former NFL players like Junior Seau and Aaron Hernandez or NHL players like Derek Boogaard. As a result, some people believe that, if their child only plays contact sports through the youth or high school level, they can't get this disease. But *CTE is not just a disease that affects professional athletes*, and some of the saddest stories involve those who are not famous. The disease has been diagnosed in athletes who only played their sport at the youth level or for just a few years in high school.[28] CTE has been diagnosed in several athletes under age twenty and many more athletes in their twenties or thirties. The youngest reported case was a seventeen-year-old boy.

Exposure to repetitive brain trauma is at least a strong risk factor, if not the key factor, for developing CTE.[29] Nearly all cases have a history of repetitive impacts. Very few CTE cases have been diagnosed in a person without a known history of repetitive impacts, though the researchers may not have been aware of impacts these individuals sustained in their lifetime.[30] Even those studies found that individuals who played contact sports, especially football, were at greater odds of having CTE. Other reported CTE cases with no known history of repetitive impacts have been questioned by experts who believe the tau in the brain was actually from a different disease, not CTE. Even if repetitive brain trauma is not necessary to develop the disease, it seems to be a major risk factor.

Anyone exposed to repetitive brain trauma could be at risk for getting CTE. Football is the sport that has been studied the most in recent years, and hundreds of football players have been diagnosed with the disease.[31] As of 2018, 147 college football programs had at least one former player diagnosed with CTE, including each member of the power five conferences. But CTE is not just a disease of football players. Cases have been diagnosed in NHL and junior hockey players, soccer players, rugby players, Australian football players, a professional BMX rider, entertainment wrestlers, and boxers.[32] CTE has also been diagnosed in nonathletes, including military veterans with blast exposure and a victim of domestic abuse.[33] The brain doesn't know what hits it; it just feels the force of the impact. So any source of repetitive brain trauma could cause the disease.

The total amount of repetitive brain trauma matters. Though there is no known threshold of impacts needed to develop the disease, the likelihood of developing CTE has been correlated with the number of years football players played the game. A 2019 study found that for every additional year of football played, the odds of having CTE increased by 30 percent.[34] Those who played the game for fifteen years or more were ten times more likely to be diagnosed with CTE, though some who played that long did not develop the disease. On the other end of the spectrum, those who played just four years or less were ten times less likely to be diagnosed with the disease, though it was diagnosed in some who played less than four years.

There is no evidence that one or even a few concussions without additional exposure can lead to CTE.[35] The risk may be influenced by a spectrum of impact intensity, frequency, and quantity. Sustaining a lower number of high-force, concussive impacts may have a similar risk to sustaining a high number of low-force impacts. Concussions alone shouldn't be the sole worry. Up to 16 percent of individuals diagnosed with CTE had never been diagnosed with a concussion, but they typically played positions known to be exposed to a high number of impacts. It seems that sustaining repetitive brain trauma is enough to cause CTE without ever having a concussion, and this is supported by evidence of changes in the brain after one season of repetitive subconcussive impacts in contact sports. It's important to keep in mind, though, that many athletes don't report their concussions. It's likely that some of the athletes with CTE but no diagnosed concussion had actually sustained concussions that went unreported and undiagnosed.

While repetitive brain trauma can lead to CTE, not everyone exposed to these repeated hits goes on to develop the disease. There are likely other risk factors that make someone more or less susceptible. This could include substance abuse, inflammation, or other factors that cause stress to typical body physiological processes.[36] Certain genes could affect the risk that someone may get the disease or hasten the onset of disease symptoms, and research is investigating several potential candidates. Some genes may be related to CTE risk, while different genetic factors may actually make a person less likely to develop the disease.

At this time, the vast majority of CTE cases have been diagnosed in males. The number of cases diagnosed in females is in the single digits.[37] Women are at risk of repetitive head impacts in soccer, hockey, rugby, competitive cheerleading, and many other sports. While it's possible that females have some genetic or physiological resistance to developing the disease, there are other more likely explanations. First, it's likely that the disease has sadly been overlooked in some women, such as victims of domestic violence. Far more research is needed on how CTE affects the millions of victims of domestic violence each year. A second factor is the historical lack of opportunity for females to play sports. Title IX was passed in 1972, which mandated that federally funded educational institutions provide females with the same opportunities as males, including in athletics.[38] After this, options for girls and women in sports increased immensely, but it still took a long time for women's sports to reach today's levels. The first generation of women with more widespread participation in sports that regularly exposed them to repetitive impacts are just now reaching middle age, which is when symptoms of CTE most commonly begin to appear. It is possible that we will begin to see more females diagnosed with CTE within the coming decades.

Based on our current knowledge, it is reasonable to say a ten-year NFL veteran has higher odds of getting CTE than someone who only played four years of youth football. Yet we can't say for sure if either of these players will or won't get the disease. We don't know what exactly qualifies a person exposed to repetitive impacts as being at high or low risk, and I caution against making claims about risk in either direction about an individual or group. These claims have fueled arguments that the issue is being overblown and youth sports are completely safe, leaving some children exposed to repetitive brain trauma. These claims have also led some people to believe that their symptoms were absolutely from CTE and they had no hope for their future when that wasn't true. In some devastating cases, it played a role in them taking their own lives. A survey of NCAA Division I football players found that one in ten predicted that they would develop dementia or CTE from concussions, despite the fact that we don't know how common the disease is in college players.[39] The truth is, repetitive brain trauma in contact sports at all levels of play, from youth and recreational levels to the pros, can lead to the development of this neurodegenerative disease, and we need to accept that the risk is real. Yet many athletes don't get the disease, and we have a lot to learn about how common it is in contact sport athletes.

CTE AND PARTICIPATION IN YOUTH SPORTS

Could playing a contact sport in youth put a child at risk of developing CTE, even if they don't go on to play in high school or college? Should concern about CTE influence the decision about whether or not to let a child play a contact sport?

CTE is a valid concern. In some people, the neurodegenerative process starts early, though we don't know exactly why. CTE can happen even in teenagers or after only playing at the youth or high school levels.[40] The risk seems very low if a youth athlete only plays the sport for a few years. Yet incurring repetitive impacts at a young age may hasten the onset of CTE symptoms in those who do develop the disease.

A 2018 BU CTE Center study examined 246 former football players whose brains were donated for study, 211 of whom were diagnosed with CTE. Over 60 percent of the CTE cases were in former NFL players, but around one-third only played through the youth, high school, or college level.[41] The age they started playing tackle football was related to the age at which their symptoms began to show even after accounting for the number of years and decade in which they played. Those who started tackling before age twelve had an onset of symptoms about thirteen years earlier than those who began playing at an older age. For every one year younger they began tackling, the average onset of symptoms was about two and a half years earlier.

It is important to understand that this does *not* mean they were at a higher risk for getting CTE because they played at a younger age. Unfortunately, when this study came out, the media often interpreted it that way, but that is not the case. The amount of CTE pathology in the brain was not associated with the age they started playing football in this study, meaning that playing at a younger age did not make the disease worse. Another study found no increased odds of having CTE in those who started playing before age twelve.[42] There is no evidence to suggest that exposure to repetitive impacts through contact sports at a young age, when the brain is rapidly maturing, increases the risk of developing CTE or the severity of the disease, only the onset of disease symptoms. From what we know now, it seems that a child who played tackle football from ages eight to twelve would have a similar risk for CTE as a child who played from ages fourteen to eighteen.

However, those who start playing a sport at an earlier age tend to play for more years. Take two offensive linemen who both play football through their senior year of high school. One started playing in fifth grade while the other didn't start playing until their freshman year of high school. Though they both played the four years in high school, the first player experienced four more years of hits prior to that, likely incurring hundreds if not thousands of additional impacts over that time. Having more years of exposure to repetitive impacts increases the likelihood of developing CTE. As a result, starting to play at a younger age likely increases the risk for developing CTE by increasing career exposure to repetitive subconcussive impacts.

Taken together, it seems that sustaining repetitive brain trauma at a young age does not influence the development or level of disease of CTE, but it does affect how early symptoms show in someone who does get CTE. How is that possible? Our brain is incredibly resilient. Even with a remarkable amount of damage and neuron loss, the brain will do everything it can to compensate and function normally for as long as it can. Eventually there aren't enough neurons left and connections in the brain to sustain normal function. Once the symptoms start to show, a great deal of disease is already present. As with accelerated aging, environmental factors such as alcohol dependence, cigarette smoking, and HIV-related inflammation have been linked to an onset of Alzheimer's disease symptoms at a younger age.[43] Similarly, disrupted development from repetitive impacts in childhood could leave a person who started early with less cognitive reserve, or having "less gas in the tank" in adulthood, compared to someone who started a contact sport at an older age. If they both go on to develop CTE anyway, the athlete who began playing, and incurring repetitive impacts, at an earlier age would likely be younger when their CTE symptoms began to show.

In contrast, increasing cognitive reserve, or putting extra gas in the tank, can help stave off the onset of CTE symptoms. In one study of diagnosed CTE, only two individuals with stage II CTE had no symptoms, one in their forties and another in their eighties. Both were successful professionals with advanced graduate degrees.[44] Another CTE Center study examined cognitive reserve and CTE symptoms onset in former NFL players who died at an average age of sixty-five.[45] Those who had a higher cognitive reserve, based on having a professional, technical, or managerial job after their time in the league, had an onset of symptoms nearly eleven years later than those with a lower cognitive reserve. This is why it is so important to exercise both your brain and your body throughout life.

THE SKEPTICS, THE RISK, AND THE REALITY

Despite all we have learned, there are some who are skeptical that CTE can be caused by repetitive subconcussive impacts. Though plausible theories exist, we don't know the exact biological mechanisms that lead from repetitive brain trauma to the development of CTE pathology. Yet a lack of complete understanding doesn't mean we don't know enough now to say that exposure to repetitive impacts is at least a substantial risk factor for CTE. And with millions of young athletes exposed to these repetitive impacts, it is a public health concern.

Some cite the few cases of CTE diagnosed in those with no known history of repetitive impacts as proof that the impacts do not cause the disease. Even if CTE can develop in a person who does not have exposure to repetitive brain trauma, it doesn't make repetitive brain trauma any less of a risk factor for developing the disease.[46] Other factors, such as alcohol abuse or performance enhancing drugs, very well could contribute to CTE development, but it seems unlikely they would be a primary cause given that teen athletes have been diagnosed with the disease. Even if those factors could cause the disease, that has no relevance for repetitive impacts being a risk factor. Lung cancer has many causes, including genetic factors, radon exposure, and exposure to asbestos. Of course, one of the biggest risk factors for developing lung cancer is smoking. The fact that those other causes exist doesn't make smoking any safer or any less of a substantial risk factor. One thing being dangerous doesn't automatically make something else safe. Yet not everyone will get the disease. Not all smokers get lung cancer, and not all NFL players get CTE. A lack of disease in someone exposed to decades of repetitive impacts doesn't mean those impacts are safe either.

WHAT DOES THIS MEAN FOR YOUTH CONTACT SPORT ATHLETES?

The risk of developing CTE is likely low in a child who only plays a few years of youth contact sports, but the risk that these repetitive head impacts could disrupt normal brain development exists regardless of whether or not someone goes on to develop the disease. We should be at least equally if not more concerned about altering the trajectory of our children's brain development as we are about children developing CTE from youth sports. Though impacts in youth do not seem to cause CTE, they do seem to influence how early the disease symptoms begin and progress if the disease develops. And playing at a younger age likely means more lifetime impacts and, in turn, a higher risk of developing CTE. I caution parents against holding a child out of sports in general simply out of fears of brain trauma and CTE. Though we still have much to learn, there are ways we can minimize the risk of any long-term consequences of repetitive head impacts in youth sports.

Part III

Bad Arguments for Maintaining the Status Quo in Youth Contact Sports

Chapter Nine

Why the Argument That "Other Sports Are Dangerous Too" Is a Bad One

Riding a bike or a skateboard are not known to cause hundreds of impacts to the head in a year.
—Chris Nowinski, cofounder and CEO of the Concussion Legacy Foundation[1]

"Most concussions in kids happen while riding a bike."
"You can get in a car accident or fall and get a concussion."
"Girls' soccer is really the most dangerous sport for the brain."

These are common arguments I hear from those defending youth contact sports in the discussion of brain trauma and potential long-term consequences. They are most commonly used with youth football in the United States, and with rugby, Australian football, and soccer in other countries around the world. I once heard a coach ask, when talking about the safety of organized youth football, "Would you rather they be playing a pickup game on the streets?" Okay, so maybe a neighborhood game of tackle football on concrete is dangerous, but that doesn't make the organized version with helmets and coaches safe for the brain either.

The arguments are centered around three main thoughts: other common childhood activities for kids can result in brain trauma, there is risk in everyday life, and other common sports are dangerous for the brain too. Supporters of youth contact sports often use these excuses to justify why their sport is safe to play. This chapter will address these arguments and discuss why, although they might seem reasonable, they say little about the actual risk of consequences for the brains of youth athletes.

TWO THINGS CAN BE DANGEROUS AT THE SAME TIME

Imagine you have an eight-year-old child who enjoys juggling. He comes to you one day and asks if he could juggle your butcher knives, like in a YouTube video he watched. When you say, "No, it's too dangerous," he replies, "But it's safer than juggling chainsaws like they did in the other video!" Well, sure, he may be right, but that doesn't make juggling butcher knives a safe activity for an eight-year-old (or anyone, for that matter). The point is, one activity being safer than another has no bearing on the safety of the other activity. Two things can be dangerous at the same time.

One of the most common arguments I hear is that riding a bicycle is more dangerous and results in more concussions each year than youth contact sports. In 2016, over 8.6 million children ages six to twelve reported riding a bike at least once per year, which is far more than the number of children reported to have played football, hockey, soccer, and rugby combined in the United States.[2] With so many more kids riding bikes than playing football, it would make sense that the overall number of concussions from riding a bike would also be higher than the number of concussions from playing football. But the data simply doesn't support this.

From 2010 to 2016, about 26,000 children under the age of eighteen visited an emergency department each year for a traumatic brain injury, including concussions, that happened while riding a bike.[3] That seems like a lot of kids, but the same report found that brain injuries occurred while playing football in over 53,000 children per year who visited the emergency department. The ten- to fourteen-year-old group had the highest number of reported traumatic brain injuries, with 32.6 percent occurring while playing football compared to just 9.4 percent while riding a bicycle. The brain-injury-related emergency department visits were similar between football and bicycling for five- to nine-year-old males, while the rate in fifteen- to seventeen-year-old males from football was more than four times that of bicycling per year. Not all kids who sustain a concussion go to the emergency department. Many of these injuries are managed by athletic trainers and team physicians in the sports setting. That is rarely the case for concussions from bike accidents. If cases managed by providers outside of the emergency department were included, the football rates would likely be much higher compared to those for riding a bike. This is just one study, but its massive scale, with an average of 283,000 children per year across sixty-six hospitals nationwide, lends strong credibility to the findings.

Even if we were to consider the risk of sustaining a concussion to be similar between riding a bike and playing football, there is a critical difference between these activities: *how many times does your child hit their head on an average bike ride?* I hope the answer is zero. Repetitive hits to the head are an inherent part of contact sports, and they are particularly high in sports like football and rugby. Hits like the ones that happen every play, with every tackle and every collision, are not part of a typical bike ride. And as you have learned, these subconcussive hits have consequences for the developing brain. When a concussion does happen on a bike ride, it is because of an accident. But concussions happen all the time in contact sports from routine plays that are a normal part of the game. Of course, no player is trying to get a concussion, but the plays that cause them are not accidents.

This same idea is true for other activities of daily life. Some advocates for contact sports for young kids argue that life has risks, and the benefits outweigh the risks with these sports. Sure, we do risky things every day. Simply riding in a car is dangerous. You could slip and fall on an icy sidewalk or wet floor. But how many times do you hit your head on a typical car ride or while you are walking? My husband sustained a concussion emptying the dishwasher when he hit his head on a cupboard door. Does that mean he's never going to empty the dishwasher again? Of course not. But he doesn't hit his head multiple times every time he empties the dishwasher either. Repetitive brain trauma is not a typical part of everyday life.

Riding in a car poses risks. But we have to get from point A to point B in our lives every day, and for most people that involves a car. The benefits outweigh the risks. Participation in sports in which repetitive impacts are built into the game will obviously greatly increase the chance that our brain will sustain damage as it is jostled around within our skull. We don't *have to* play a specific form of a sport that involves ramming our heads into each other or a ball, especially in childhood when the brain is rapidly developing. That is optional, and the benefits of sports can be gained in different ways.

MULTIPLE SPORTS CARRY A HIGH RISK FOR BRAIN TRAUMA

Supporters of a given contact sport often argue that concussions and repetitive impacts are common in other sports, too, as a way to draw attention away from the dangers of their sport. Those supporting football say we should be worried about hockey or soccer. Those supporting hockey and soccer say their sports are fine because football is far worse. This happens at different levels of play as well, with many saying that kids don't hit that hard, so we should be more worried about the high school and college players. As you have read, that just isn't true. Ultimately, this attempt to divert attention away from the dangers of a given sport ignores one important point: one sport being safer than another doesn't make either sport safe for the brain.

Soccer is the number one sport-related cause of concussions in girls.[4] Those who support youth tackle football often cite research that found a higher concussion rate in girls' soccer than in football as a reason we should be more worried about girls' soccer.[5] But that one study is in the minority. As described in chapter 5, the vast majority of studies show football has the highest concussion rate of all youth and high school organized sports in the United States. Still, other sports like hockey, lacrosse, wrestling, and even basketball, especially for girls, have relatively high concussion rates, and they deserve attention when it comes to concussion prevention and management as well. But it's not all about concussions. Tackle football is the sport with the greatest number of impacts in an average season as well, though hockey is not far behind. Though the data is limited, rugby likely involves a high number of impacts too.

But the risks of one sport have no bearing on how risky another sport is. Even if a few studies find hockey or girls' soccer have a slightly higher concussion rate than football, it doesn't somehow make the rate in football low. Even though football has the highest average impact exposure over a season at all levels, it doesn't make the hundreds of impacts sustained in hockey any less concerning. All of these sports need to take meaningful steps to protect the developing brains of their young athletes.

Many changes have been made to improve brain safety in sports, with several sports eliminating the primary source of brain trauma at youth levels. Football has introduced several changes, including reducing contact time in practice and emphasizing "proper" tackling technique, but leaders in the youth game haven't gone so far as to eliminate the primary source of impacts and concussions in the youth game: tackling. Without tackling and with different blocking styles, the number of impacts sustained is substantially lower in the flag version of the game, and head-to-head contact is rare.[6]

Yet, when some have proposed flag football for all youth players, a version of the game that would eliminate the primary source of impacts, many proponents of tackle football like to cite a study out of Iowa that found higher injury rates in flag football than tackle football.[7] But does this study really show that flag football is more dangerous? No, it does not. The study included 3,525 tackle football players who participated in a total of 44,164 individual events and sustained thirty concussions compared to just 219 players, 2,252 total events, and three concussions on the flag football side. Those are substantial differences between groups, which can affect the outcomes. The difference in concussion rate between flag and tackle was not statistically meaningful, and we can't draw any conclusions based on just three concussions. One accidental collision (and it would be an accident in flag football) could have caused two concussions, completely skewing the data. When compared to other studies, both the overall injury rate and concussion rate in the tackle football players in this study are substantially lower than the rates in other studies of youth tackle football,[8] which may be due to a lack of recognition, lack of recording, or just a random lucky year. The flag football concussion rate was also lower than concussion rates in most other studies of youth tackle football. Of course, one study alone is never enough to draw conclusions, and future research will tell us more about injuries in flag football.

CONCUSSIONS AND SUBCONCUSSIVE IMPACTS ARE CONCERNING IN ANY SPORT

In the arguments for maintaining contact sports as they currently are, the comparisons of risk to other sports or activities just don't hold water. We take small risks every day. Some are immediate risks, like riding in a car. Some are long-term risks, like smoking or consuming a poor diet that can lead to disease. I've even heard the argument from youth tackle football supporters that "Sugar is bad for kids. Does that mean we are going to ban sugar too?" Well, consuming too much sugar can have substantial negative impacts on our health, so we should be concerned about that as well. But what does that have to do with brain safety in football? Absolutely nothing. More than one thing can be bad for us at the same time.

Concussions can happen in aspects of daily life and in other sports. Several contact sports can also subject kids to repetitive impacts. But the risks associated with one sport do not automatically imply that another sport is safe. We need to make all of these sports as safe as possible for our kids. They don't have to sustain these impacts. We can provide opportunities and choose to have kids play versions of these sports that don't involve inherent repetitive impacts than can damage their developing brain.

Chapter Ten

Why Helmets and Other Technology Won't Solve the Problem

We parents do everything possible to keep our kids healthy, to allow our kids to reach their full potential. . . . Then those same parents drop a kid off at a field, tell them to put this big helmet and mask on their head . . . those big plastic helmets make them kind of unsteady and at the same time think that they're invincible; they don't feel little hits over and over again.
—Robert Stern, PhD, director of clinical research, CTE Center, Boston University School of Medicine[1]

It is widely thought that technology can help the sports world solve the concussion crisis.[2] Parents want to do everything they can to protect their children, and some have spent hundreds or even thousands of dollars on new "state-of-the-art" helmets and products that claim to "prevent concussions" or speed recovery from the injury. Coaches and leagues invest a lot of money in cutting-edge safety equipment, often requiring their athletes to use it despite a lack of evidence to support the company's claims. While this may make parents feel like the coaches or league care about their kids, these technologies often offer little, if any, real protection.

Athletes may feel more confident and better protected when they use new helmets, headgear, or other products, but this can give them a false sense of security.[3] Risk compensation happens when athletes think that equipment or other products are protecting them, so they take more risks and play more recklessly.[4] As a result, they may actually expose themselves to more danger by using the product. This occurs even with products that offer some value, like helmets, but the perceived protection is more than the actual protection. Risk compensation can be seen throughout the history of sports. For example, players began using their helmets to spear-tackle after hard-shelled helmets became popular in the 1950s.[5]

This chapter will discuss why helmets and other technology won't solve the problems associated with repetitive subconcussive impacts or concussions in youth sports. Advancements in sport safety technology have been filled with both beneficial innovations and pseudoscience. All stakeholders involved in youth sports should be cautious about buying into the hype.

HELMETS

In helmeted contact sports, like football, hockey, and lacrosse, coaches and sports organizations often claim new helmets will protect the brains of young athletes. This is, at best, an overstatement. Helmets are critically important for preventing skull fractures, and they may be able to absorb some impact force that would otherwise be transmitted to the brain. Yet claims that any helmets are "concussion proof" or can substantially reduce the risk of sustaining a concussion are untrue, misleading, or exaggerated. Concussion-proof helmets do not, and will not ever, exist, and no helmet can prevent the effects of all subconcussive impacts. Remember, you don't have to hit your head to get a concussion. A hit to the body can transmit damaging forces to the brain even if the head is not impacted. No helmet can prevent the brain from moving inside the skull.

A Brief History of Helmets in Contact Sports

Football: The first football helmet was worn in the 1893 Army–Navy game.[6] Made of leather, these helmets provided very little protection, and many players chose not to wear them. A suspension system that separated the outer padded shell from the skull was first used in 1917 and did a better job of absorbing and distributing some impact forces. They were not made mandatory for NCAA players until 1939, with the NFL following suit one year later. The first plastic helmet was created in 1939, but they were not mass-produced until after World War II.[7] Hard-shell helmets were originally designed with the goal of preventing potentially deadly skull fractures and brain bleeds.[8] Players felt protected by these new helmets, and it became more common for athletes to use their head as a weapon.[9] When face masks were introduced in the 1950s, players didn't have to worry as much about broken noses or other facial injuries.[10] Coaches encouraged aggressive behavior, as helmet-first impacts could produce crushing blows that would lead to a turnover. Helmets have continued to improve over the last several decades with new innovative designs and materials. With those improvements, risk compensation continues to be an issue as players feel their brains are more protected than they actually are.

Hockey: The first hockey helmets were worn in the 1920s, but it wasn't until the 1970s that their use rose substantially in the NHL.[11] Even goalie masks were not worn in the league until 1959. Many players considered playing without a helmet or mask a sign of toughness.[12] While few players wore helmets in 1970, nearly two-thirds wore them by 1980. Helmets became mandatory for all new players entering the NHL in 1979. Though some veterans also saw the value in this safety equipment, there were many holdouts. Craig MacTavish retired in 1997 as the last NHL player to play without a helmet.[13]

Lacrosse: The use of leather lacrosse helmets was first documented in the 1928 Olympics.[14] The bucket-style helmet with a suspension system and hard outer shell grew in popularity in the 1980s. Lacrosse helmets have continued to evolve since then, with sleek designs and lighter materials.[15] Helmets are not worn in women's lacrosse, which is played with different rules than the men's game.[16] Female players at all levels are required to wear eye protection, while headgear (US Lacrosse does not call them helmets) is allowed but not required. Headgear made specifically for the women's game was only first developed in the 2010s. Its effectiveness for injury prevention is currently being evaluated.

Standards Organizations: Despite advancements in helmets, too many boys and young men, more than thirty per year, were still dying on the football field in the 1960s and early 1970s.[17] In 1970 the National Operating Committee on Standards for Athletic Equipment (NOCSAE) was formed with a goal of reducing injuries in sport.[18] NOCSAE worked to develop standards for laboratory testing that would evaluate the ability of a helmet to prevent catastrophic injuries like skull fractures by absorbing a sufficient amount of energy from an impact. In

1971 the American Society for Testing and Materials (ASTM) also began developing methods for testing football helmets, followed by hockey helmets and other headgear in the following years.[19] After the development of NOCSAE and ASTM standards, the annual incidence of fatalities dropped substantially to about a quarter of what it had been in years before the standards were implemented.

How Do Helmets Work?

Hard-shell helmets, like those worn in football, hockey, lacrosse, and baseball or softball, can be very effective at protecting against skull fractures.[20] They are also capable of absorbing and redistributing a limited amount of impact forces, having some influence on concussion risk. Still, no helmet can lessen these forces enough to prevent all concussions or consequences of subconcussive impacts. The hard shell and face mask of helmets deflect impacts, redistribute forces, and protect the skull.[21] The padding underneath functions to absorb energy and slow the impact. When we slow the impact, we can slow the acceleration, which helps with linear acceleration. However, when the impact time is longer, the head will rotate more. Though rotational acceleration may be lower, rotating for more time means rotating a farther distance, which may result in more damage to the brain's white matter.

Most helmets have to meet standards set by either NOCSAE or ASTM. The NOCSAE standard is set based on a severity index. A helmet passes the test with a severity index less than 1200.[22] The lower the score, the better. However, this does not consider rotational acceleration, only linear acceleration. The biomechanical firm Biokinetics found that helmets way below 1200, even below a score of 300, will still allow for at least a 50 percent chance of sustaining a concussion at the acceleration tested. These standards were never intended to evaluate concussion prevention, and their results should not be interpreted that way.

How Well Do Helmets Work?

A few studies have examined concussion rates among different helmets. While one study found a difference between two helmet models from the same company,[23] other studies have found little or no difference in concussion rates between helmets from different companies.[24] Even reconditioned helmets provide similar protection compared to new helmets, though older helmets that have not been reconditioned may increase the risk of concussions.

Of course, helmet companies need to sell helmets to make money, and they sometimes interpret research in a way that benefits them. Riddell did just that with a 2006 study.[25] They claimed the study found that athletes who wore their Revolution helmet had a 31 percent lower risk of sustaining a concussion, but they misrepresented the results. The next paragraph is a little math heavy. If you're not into that, feel free to skip to the last sentence for the conclusion.

In the study, 7.6 percent of athletes wearing other helmets and 5.3 percent of athletes wearing the Revolution helmet sustained a concussion. Comparing these two percentages to each other, 5.3 is 69 percent of 7.6. This means the Revolution was 31 percent better than other helmets in the study. But over 92 percent of athletes in both groups did not sustain a concussion. The absolute risk in the study is 7.6 percent minus 5.3 percent. This means the Revolution helmet only decreased the overall risk of sustaining a concussion by 2.3 percentage points, substantially smaller than what Riddell was claiming. The researchers voiced their disagreement publicly, warning Riddell that they were misinterpreting the results. The absolute value provides a more realistic view of the ability of the helmet to protect the brain, but Riddell continued to cite the exaggerated number.

This wasn't the first claim made by Riddell that their helmets could reduce concussions, and it wasn't the first time they were called out for overstating the protective effect of a helmet. Multiple lawsuits, including one involving thousands of former NFL players, were filed against Riddell as a result of these claims, citing that the company had misled and inadequately warned users of the potential risk of concussion that came with wearing the Revolution helmet.[26]

Overstatements of protection don't just happen with football helmets. For example, Reebok-CCM claimed its hockey helmets could prevent concussions.[27] They had to abandon their marketing campaign due to a lack of evidence to back up their claims. When companies make these claims for helmets in any sport, many parents and athletes will rush out to buy them despite the cost and lack of evidence that they can actually prevent concussions.

Engineers at Virginia Tech have developed ratings for helmets and headgear used in tackle and flag football, baseball, softball, bicycling, hockey, and soccer.[28] They test the helmets and headgear based on the biomechanics of impacts known to be common in the sport the helmet is used for. You can find current ratings on their website: https://helmet.beam.vt.edu/index.html.

Testing showed that most brands and styles of football helmets provide similar protection for the brain. In the 2020 ratings, only two helmets rated less than five stars. Despite similar ratings, cost differences can be staggering. For example, the fifth-ranked Xenith X2E+ helmet costs $289.00, while the sixth-ranked Riddell Precision-FIT helmet costs a whopping $1,700.00. Three of the top four helmets cost nearly $1,000. That's $700 more than the $289.00 model for helmets that essentially provide the same level of protection. The researchers clearly state that any helmet with a five-star rating is recommended, regardless of the exact score. Any differences in safety provided between helmets of the same rating is minimal.

Children experience different accelerations than older players due to their larger head compared to their body size, and more impacts happen with falls at the youth level.[29] These factors influence the way helmets for children should be made and tested. Virginia Tech released helmet ratings for youth football in 2019. Their testing standards were the first designed based on the nature of impacts in ten- to fourteen-year-old football players, rather than adult impact biomechanics. The majority of youth football helmets receive a five-star rating, and like the helmets for older players, the cost is *not* an indication of quality. As of 2020, the third-ranked Xenith Youth X2E+ helmet receives a five-star rating and costs $199.00. The sixth-ranked Schutt Youth F7 helmet also has five stars but sells for $569.95.

In contrast to football helmets, the Virginia Tech engineers found that most hockey helmets do a poor job of dissipating forces related to concussions. Only one helmet has a five-star rating, one has four stars, and three have three stars. The rest are rated from zero to two stars, suggesting they are, at best, adequate for preventing catastrophic injuries but do little if anything to dissipate potential concussive or subconcussive forces.

Soft-shell helmets have come on the market in recent years. One type goes on top of hard-shell football helmets. They are made of a soft foam material, and their makers claim that they can dissipate and absorb more energy with impacts. However, research has shown that they do little to reduce impact accelerations, and they can't stop the brain from moving in the skull.[30] Soft-shell flag football helmets are becoming more popular as more kids are playing that version of the game.

Virginia Tech has created ratings for these helmets as well, and several are rated four or five stars. However, the same cautions apply: though they may provide some benefit, they will not prevent all concussions or subconcussive forces.

It's important to point out that all of the helmets and headgear are tested in the laboratory setting, and sports aren't played in a lab. Aspects of sport play, such as the exact impact location, anticipation of the impact, the strength and sizes of players in the collision, and more, make every hit unique. That means the lab setting cannot possibly predict and test for every impact. The lab can be incredibly valuable for learning about the biomechanical capabilities of different types of helmets and headgear. If the equipment doesn't work well in the lab, it is unlikely that it will be effective on the field or ice. However, there is no guarantee that something that performs better in the lab will actually make a meaningful difference in the practice or game setting.

OTHER HEADGEAR

The soccer community is eager to find ways to reduce the risk of concussions, especially in female athletes. Some soccer coaches and organizations are promoting padded headgear for their players, though data suggests these may not be effective and may lead to risk compensation.[31] A 2019 study from the University of Wisconsin–Madison found that soccer headgear was not effective in reducing concussion rates, the severity of concussion symptoms, or the amount of time athletes were away from their sport after a concussion in high school players.[32] While specific headgear brands showed a slight trend toward being more effective than others, none made a meaningful difference in concussion rates. More research is needed, but at this time there is no clear evidence to suggest the headgear in soccer provides much protection for the brain.

Headgear use in rugby has had mixed results. While some studies have found that headgear may reduce concussions, other studies have shown no benefit.[33] A study of nearly 3,700 youth and adolescent rugby players from the under-thirteen to under-twenty age groups found no reduction in concussion rates in those who wore headgear.[34] Though the padding may be able to absorb some impact forces, it's not enough to make a meaningful impact on concussion rates.

MOUTH GUARDS

Some have proposed that mouth guards could dissipate forces with impacts to the jaw and, as a result, could be useful in reducing the risk of sustaining a concussion. Most studies have found no difference in concussion rates while wearing a mouth guard.[35] There is some, albeit limited, evidence to suggest that the type of mouth guard worn can make a difference. One study found a higher concussion rate in those who wore custom mouth guards compared to generic moldable plastic mouth guards.[36] While mouth guards are effective for preventing dental and some facial injuries, we should not rely on these to protect against concussions.

IMPACT SENSORS

Several companies have made helmets, mouth guards, headbands, and patches with accelerometers available to consumers on the commercial market. Many have triggers that alert the sidelines, often through a phone app, when a player takes a hit over a given threshold. The goal is to alert coaches, athletic trainers, or team doctors when an athlete takes a high-force impact so that the athlete can be evaluated for a potential concussion. The companies don't claim that these helmets can diagnose concussions, only that they can alert the coaches or medical staff when an athlete might be injured because they took a big hit. Some of these devices also record the overall number of impacts over a set threshold that a player sustains so that coaches and medical providers can monitor overall impacts.

While this seems like a great idea, it's not that simple. The threshold for alerting the sideline is supposed to mark the force at which the athlete is likely to have sustained a concussion.[37] Yet we don't know what hits do or don't cause a concussion. A hit early in a game that triggers a sideline evaluation may not cause a concussion. But research suggests that, after accumulating more impacts during the game or practice, a lower-magnitude hit that does not alert the sideline may actually cause a concussion.[38] If the sensors don't alert the sidelines about this lower-magnitude impact, the concussion may go undiagnosed.

These sensors aren't perfect. Both helmet and nonhelmet accelerometers can have false positive errors, meaning that they measure an impact that didn't actually happen.[39] Some may also miss impacts that really did happen, or they may not record impacts because they measure the accelerations as lower than they actually are. Though all sensors have some degree of error, the error can be much higher in nonhelmeted sensors. Error rates can be adjusted for, impacts can be verified with video, and the sensors may be useful at the group level in the research setting. However, at this time it is difficult to use this technology for individual players or individual impacts, especially in a live game or practice setting. The Virginia Tech engineers are in the process of evaluating the accuracy of sensors on the market for commercial use.

It's also challenging to interpret what the output of these sensors really means when the companies hold the thresholds as proprietary information. It may seem like a player has not sustained many impacts over a season based on the sensor data, but if that sensor is using a threshold of 30 or 40 g, it may be missing the majority of impacts the athlete sustained. Even if we do know the acceleration threshold, we don't know if there is a threshold of repetitive impacts in a game, season, or career over which the risk of long-term consequences is increased or under which is sure to be safe. Someday we may understand what that threshold is, and we may be able to implement a hit count, similar to a pitch count in baseball, where we monitor athletes and remove them if they sustained too many impacts in a practice or game. However, our knowledge and technology just aren't there yet.

While these helmets may give coaches and medical providers some information, the information may be misleading or may not be meaningful. This technology is important and constantly improving, and it is likely that someday these devices will be immensely useful. As we learn more about the biomechanics of concussions and the number of impacts over an event, season, or career that can lead to short- or long-term consequences, the sensors may become powerful tools for brain safety in sports. However, right now, even if we had accurate data, we don't have the ability to interpret that data in a useful way for an individual athlete.

OTHER PRODUCTS: SCIENCE AND PSEUDOSCIENCE

Nearly everyone involved in contact sports at all levels would like a quick fix that will appease fears and solve the problems associated with concussions and subconcussive impacts. Many companies claim their products will do just that, and they often target those involved in youth sports. [40] From special chocolate milk, to concussion water, to special neck-strengthening equipment, companies claim their products protect against concussions and subconcussive impacts or speed recovery from the injury without much if any validated scientific evidence that they work. Though these companies might start with good intentions, they often overstate the effectiveness of their product. They convince professional athletes to promote and sometimes invest in their products, like Russel Wilson and the fortified water he claims (without scientific evidence) can prevent concussions. [41] Youth athletes want to be like the superstars they watch on TV, so they often want to use the products that they see the superstars promoting.

One device that has made claims to prevent concussions in recent years is the jugular compression collar. It is referred to as an anticoncussion product in studies sponsored by the company that makes it. [42] The collar was inspired in part by the anatomy of woodpeckers, which use a muscle to put pressure on their jugular vein as they are pecking. [43] This is thought to limit blood flow away from the brain, increasing the pressure inside the skull to prevent the brain from moving much within the cranium. The scientists became interested in woodpeckers because it was thought that they endure thousands of impacts without sustaining brain damage. However, these birds have developed many adaptations for hitting their heads repeatedly as a natural part of their existence. And, as it turns out, they may get CTE too. A 2018 study found tau around blood vessels and in the white matter pathways of the brains of woodpeckers. [44]

Even if the jugular compression method is helpful for woodpeckers, humans are not woodpeckers. We don't have the additional adaptations that woodpeckers have in our skull. We have to consider if increasing pressure within our skull by increasing the blood in and around the brain is actually safe for a human, especially children or adolescents with a developing brain. This is literally changing the dynamics of blood flow in the brain. Parents, coaches, and athletes should be cautious and wait until much more independent research is conducted to conclude whether or not this is safe and more than minimally effective to use. Even if this device does have a small helpful effect, it cannot prevent all concussions, and subconcussive impacts could still take a toll over time.

You may have heard of programs or athletes purchasing neck-strengthening equipment aimed at preventing concussions. In theory, this should be helpful, but the evidence is inconsistent. Some studies have found that athletes with lower neck strength or imbalance in their neck muscles are more prone to higher head accelerations and may be at greater risk for concussions.[45] However, studies of hockey, soccer, and football players found no influence of neck strength on head accelerations.[46] Other research found only a minimal relationship between neck strength and concussion risk in young female athletes.[47] Neck strength alone is not enough to prevent high head accelerations, especially with unanticipated impacts when the athlete is unable to tense their neck and core muscles to prepare for contact.

Coaches and youth sports organizations often promote products for their athletes as well, such as the omega-3 fatty acid supplement promoted by Pop Warner Little Scholars claiming to help keep the brain healthy. Promoting devices or products for children or adolescents to use with minimal if any research in that age group can be irresponsible and dangerous. Most products have little if any benefit. At best, they result in a loss of money. At worst, there could be other side effects. Parents, guardians, and coaches should be cautious and do their research before giving any of these products to youth athletes.

CAN PROTECTIVE EQUIPMENT BE IMPROVED TO HELP PREVENT CONCUSSIONS?

In laboratory settings, researchers continue to study ways to improve helmets and other safety equipment. It's possible that a helmet or headgear designed with padding targeted for vulnerable impact positions could better dissipate impact forces and increase safety. Many helmet companies are using innovative designs to try to dampen rotational accelerations.

Though this safety equipment may help to some degree, no helmet, headgear, or device will prevent all concussions or subconcussive impacts. The brain will continue to move in the skull, even if the head itself is not impacted. The bottom line is this: do your research and understand the limitations before spending your hard-earned money on products claiming to protect the brain. The best way to protect the brain will always be to avoid these impacts altogether.

Chapter Eleven

Why "Safer Than Ever" May Not Be Safe Enough

We see euphemisms like, "Safer than ever," and vague notions of safer tackling, whatever that means. I made 400-something tackles at Wisconsin and never discovered how to do it safely. Those are company lines. It's PR.

—Chris Borland, former linebacker, Wisconsin Badgers and
San Francisco 49ers[1]

Over the past decade, rule changes have been made in contact sports with a goal of reducing concussions and overall head impacts. Some sports have implemented bans on aspects of their game before a certain age, and other sports have tweaked rules and emphasized "proper" techniques for high-risk maneuvers. Concussion education efforts have increased substantially over the last decade too. As a result of all of these changes, as well as both real and perceived advances in equipment, some people argue that contact sports are safer than they have ever been.

While the primary goal of these rule changes has been to improve safety for athletes in these sports, another key goal has been to convince parents and athletes that the sports are safe to play. This has been particularly evident in football, where participation in the United States has declined considerably at both the youth and high school levels, in part due to fears of brain injuries.[2] The NFL has gone to great lengths to convince parents, especially mothers, that the game is safe for their boys and girls to play.[3] They air commercials touting the changes that have been made to the game and new safety equipment. Some commercials have mothers of NFL players talking about safety. NFL teams hold safety clinics for moms to show them the "safe" tackling technique. They have spun, selectively chosen, and misrepresented research in the process. Still, some parents rely on the NFL as a trusted source of information on safety in football. But is the game really safer than ever? And is safer than ever safe enough?

In this chapter I will discuss changes that have been made to improve safety in contact sports as well as research on how effective those changes have been. It is important to look at this research with a critical eye. The headlines only tell a small part of the story, and it may only be the part of the story that a league or sport organization wants you to hear.

CATASTROPHIC INJURIES AND FATALITIES IN SPORTS

Catastrophic injuries and fatalities have declined substantially over the past century, and in that regard, contact sports are safer than ever. In some sports, these incidents have never been high, but for football, there was a lot of room for improvement. By the early 1900s football had been abolished at several universities because too many boys were dying on the field.[4] President Theodore Roosevelt was a football fan, and despite growing concern, he wanted the game to continue. He initiated a meeting with leadership from several universities that eventually resulted in the creation of the Intercollegiate Athletic Association, which became the NCAA in 1910. While the situation improved after the NCAA was established, football still had a long way to go. Helmet standards and the ban on spear tackles have helped fatalities per year fall into the single digits, and catastrophic spinal cord injuries have also declined. The lowest catastrophic injury rates in football occurred in the late 1990s, and they have risen slightly since that time.[5]

Though the rate of catastrophic injuries and fatalities is slightly higher in hockey at the high school level, the overall numbers are quite low, with only four fatal and fourteen nonfatal (like spinal cord injuries) incidents occurring from 1982 to 2018.[6] Football saw 137 fatalities and 411 nonfatal catastrophic injuries over the same time. More kids play football than hockey, but these are still high numbers. Rugby has the greatest risk of catastrophic and fatal injuries among popular sports internationally, with rates higher than football in most studies.[7] Still, these injuries are rare in all sports. The risk is still present, but when it comes to fatalities and life-altering injuries, these sports are much safer than they were several decades ago.

WHY WE NEED TO STUDY ANY SAFETY-RELATED RULE CHANGES

Rule changes are implemented with a specific outcome in mind, but things don't always work out as intended. In 2017, the NCAA eliminated two-a-day practices in the preseason for all Division I Football Bowl Subdivision programs, which include the big football teams you see on TV.[8] This change seemed to be aimed, at least in part, at reducing impacts. To allow for the same number of practices, teams could start a few days earlier, spreading the practices over more total days but maintaining a three-hour limit for each practice. At the same time, the NCAA and Department of Defense had partnered for a large study of college athletes. Researchers in this Concussion Assessment, Research, and Education (CARE) Consortium study examined the effects of the preseason practice changes across five teams. The results were unexpected.

Compared to 2016, athletes sustained more impacts per hour and averaged 26 percent more overall impacts in the preseason in 2017. It's possible that the intensity of practices may have been higher when they only occurred once per day. The players may have been more aggressive because they were well rested. The coaches may have had the perception that they had less practice time, so they fit more into practice. Either way, the athletes hit more when they had the same number of practices but only one practice per day.

In 2018, the NCAA responded by decreasing the number of preseason on-field contact practices from twenty-nine to twenty-five. The CARE Consortium studied this change, too, and again, the results weren't quite what they expected.[9] The number of impacts remained roughly the same from the 2017 to the 2018 season, despite fewer practices. But this varied substantially by team, with some teams seeing large decreases in preseason impacts and one experiencing an average of 35 percent more impacts in the preseason. Longer practices and a greater practice intensity seemed to play a role in the increased hits for this team.

These studies highlight how challenging it can be to implement broad policy changes that result in the intended outcomes in sport. It's reasonable to think that reducing the number or amount of time of contact practices would result in fewer impacts. Unfortunately, it's just not that simple. Coaches may respond to reduced contact time by simply packing in more contact per minute. Regulating the intensity of practice is challenging, as it typically falls on coaches to determine the type and number of drills and amount of live play in practice.

IMPROVING SAFETY IN HOCKEY AND LACROSSE

The USA Hockey rulebook defines a legal body check as when a player hits an opposing player who has the puck with the goal of getting the puck away from the opposing player.[10] Most fans, players, and coaches agree that this action can bring energy and excitement to the game. However, checking accounts for 45 to 86 percent of injuries in youth hockey players, and it is the most common cause of concussions in the sport.[11]

In 2011, USA Hockey delayed the introduction of checking until age thirteen.[12] Checking had already been banned in Quebec, but Hockey Canada followed in 2013 with a similar rule at the national level. In this case, the rule had the intended effect. Not only did the concussion rate decline significantly after it was implemented, but the overall injury rate fell too.[13] It has been estimated that nearly five thousand concussions are prevented across Canada annually as a result of this rule. One study in the United States found a substantial decrease in the number of injuries after the checking rules were implemented, but concussions rose.[14] However, the researchers suggest this rise was likely due to substantial increases in concussion education and awareness at the same time leading to improved concussion reporting and recognition.

The rule change was accompanied by backlash and controversy. Some thought fewer boys would play the sport since they couldn't play like the pros they idolize. But registration at the youth levels has actually increased.[15] Players surveyed didn't seem to mind either. Players who entered the peewee level after the rule was implemented did not feel as strongly about the importance of checking or were more likely to want to play in a league that did not have checking.[16] In general, if they haven't started checking yet, the young players don't miss it, and they aren't as likely to feel as if they want or need to check to have fun playing hockey.[17] The game was not harmed by this new rule, and safety improved.

US Lacrosse also implemented a ban on checking for boys at the under-twelve level and below in 2017.[18] Players at the under-fourteen level are allowed to check, but checking with the intent to put the opposing player on the ground remains illegal. US Lacrosse also banned stick checking for girls at the under-eleven level and below.[19] Player contact is the main source of injury in boys' lacrosse, especially at the youth level, though checking-related injuries are low overall.[20] Research is still needed to examine the outcomes of these rule changes.

IMPROVING SAFETY IN SOCCER

In 2015, US Soccer delayed the introduction of heading at the youth level.[21] Players are not allowed to head the ball until age eleven.[22] Players ages eleven and twelve years old are limited to twenty-five headers per week. It's common for soccer players to play in multiple seasons and on multiple teams, even at the same time. Twenty-five impacts per week can add up to hundreds of impacts on the developing brain each year. There has been little research into the outcomes of delaying and limiting heading in youth soccer thus far.

Soccer associations in Scotland, England, and Northern Ireland announced a similar rule in early 2020, banning heading under age eleven, then gradually introducing the practice through age eighteen.[23] Football (soccer) Federation Australia is also reviewing youth heading policies, and more countries will likely follow.[24] These bans have not come without controversy, with some favoring teaching proper technique rather than banning the practice at young ages. Others argue that the brain is still affected even with "proper" technique, and kids can learn that aspect of soccer at an older age while focusing on other skills when they are younger.

IMPROVING SAFETY IN RUGBY AND AUSTRALIAN FOOTBALL

Both rugby and Australian football have made rule changes in recent years to improve safety in their sport. Many efforts have been aimed at reducing head contact, but enforcement of these rules has sometimes been lacking, with light punishments doing little to deter players.[25]

A study of elite rugby players investigated the effect of rules forcing players to tackle below the level of the opposing player's armpit.[26] The rule change led to significantly fewer head impacts for ballcarriers, but the concussion rate doubled in tacklers. To make the tackle below the legal line, tacklers had to bend lower, causing them to lead more with their head compared to tackling in an upright position. This is another example of why it is so important to study the effects of these rule changes to make sure the intended goals are being met.

At the youth level, rugby and Australian football have improved concussion education and management, but less has been done to prevent repetitive impacts. Both sports have touch or flag versions to introduce young athletes to the game, but the tackle version can start as young as age eight. Organizations claim that changes in these sports have greatly increased safety.[27] USA Rugby's development model touts "age appropriate development" in the game but doesn't say at what age it is safe to tackle and incur repetitive impacts.[28] Most safety measures have involved rule changes for the scrum and dangerous tackles, matching youth players by size, and education on proper tackles, scrums, and injury management. Future research will determine if these rule changes and programs have been effective.

IMPROVING SAFETY IN FOOTBALL

Parents, medical providers, educators, and other stakeholders have been concerned about the safety of football since it was first played. In the 1950s, the American Academy of Pediatrics argued that the game was too dangerous for young boys to play, and doctors called for a ban on the sport for children ages twelve or younger.[29] But those concerns became overshadowed by its growing popularity and a cultural need for a way to turn boys into men. Some believed proper supervision and medical care were the keys to safety in the sport, claiming the risks were low as long as coaches were there to oversee play and doctors were there to manage injuries. While this has been repeatedly proven untrue, that mindset continues today. Better training for coaches and supervision and training with "safe" tackling techniques have been touted as game changers in recent years, when in reality, this reliance on supervision will likely fall short again.

In recent decades, changes have been made across all levels of football with a goal of improving safety and reducing concussions and subconcussive impacts. Targeting rules aim to protect defenseless players from forcible contact to the head or neck. The Ivy league has been at the forefront of positive changes in the NCAA. In 2016 the league eliminated full contact from practices.[30] They implemented new rules to increase touchbacks on kickoffs leading to an 81 percent decline in concussions on kickoffs. The NFL has also enacted similar rules to encourage more touchbacks and decrease injury, including moving kickoffs up five yards and moving touchbacks from the twenty to the twenty-five yard line.[31] These changes led to 35 percent fewer concussions on kickoffs during the 2018 NFL season.[32]

Changes have also been made at the youth and high school levels. USA Football has introduced rookie tackle football as a beginner's version of the game.[33] It involves fewer players on smaller fields, no punts or kickoffs, and no three-point stance. Yet players in rookie tackle are still tackling, and therefore still incurring repetitive brain trauma. No research exists yet to show whether or not this new form of the game is actually safer than traditional youth football.

USA Football has also introduced their football development model.[34] The program is designed to reduce contact, promote age- and skill-appropriate play, and slowly introduce and develop football skills. Much of this model is great. They emphasize development of the whole person, participating in multiple sports, and keeping the game fun. Coaches are taught to keep the mental and emotional development of the child based on their age in mind with their coaching strategies. It even provides some guidance for progressing athletes through different skills and describes non-contact, limited-contact, and contact versions of the game. However, nowhere in this model does it say at what age it is developmentally appropriate for a child to start tackling and sustaining repetitive brain trauma. In that regard, the development model falls short.

Other changes have occurred in the youth and high school game. Some have been successful, while others haven't made the substantial impact that leagues had hoped for. Researchers and sport-safety advocates have questioned whether the changes have gone far enough. What other changes have been made, and is football really safer than ever?

Tackling Technique

A big part of the claim that football is safer than ever comes from the focus on "proper tackling technique."[35] Some programs are promoting rugby-style tackling, which emphasizes "taking the head out of the game" and leading with the shoulder instead. Rugby players typically don't wear helmets, so if they lead with their head, it hurts. It's also common for players to be told to "see what you hit," or to have their head up when colliding with another player. Hitting an opponent with the top of the head increases the risk of both concussions and spinal cord injuries. This isn't a new concept though. Players have been told to "see what you hit" for decades.

Supported by the NFL, USA Football implemented its Heads Up Football educational program in 2013 to improve safety in youth football and assure parents that it was safe to let their child play the game.[36] Heads Up Tackling is a key feature of the program, but not everyone agrees that "proper" or "safe" tackling really exists. Former Wisconsin Badger and San Francisco 49er linebacker Chris Borland, who retired after just one year in the league due to concerns over brain trauma, has stated that, despite having made hundreds of tackles in his career, he hasn't learned how to tackle in a safe way.[37] Other former college and NFL players emphasize that teaching technique may be fine in low-speed drills on the practice field, but it often goes out the window in the high-speed practice and game settings. It's impossible to anticipate exactly what other players on the field will do, and a tackler will often do whatever it takes to get the ballcarrier to the ground. The program has been described as a PR stunt and marketing ploy by some. According to ESPN, former ten-year NFL quarterback Jake Plummer called it "propaganda to try to convince [kids and parents] it's safe."[38]

Researchers have studied the effects the Heads Up Football program has had on impacts and concussion rates in youth football, and that has added to the controversy. In February of 2015, USA Football used preliminary data showing significantly fewer injuries and concussions in leagues that used the Heads Up program to promote the program and the safety of youth football.[39] However, this data was preliminary, and when the actual study was published, the outcomes were quite different.[40] The study included leagues for players from five to fifteen years old. The only positive finding was that eleven- to fifteen-year-old players in both the Heads Up Football program *and* a Pop Warner program, which limits contact practice time, had a lower concussion rate than those in neither of these programs. The programs did not affect concussion rates in the five- to ten-year-old group, and involvement in only the Heads Up Football program did not influence concussion rates in any group.

In another study, those who participated in the Heads Up Football program incurred fewer impacts in practice than those not in the program. The impacts sustained in games remained similar between groups.[41] This is an important step in the right direction, but it's not clear if a few less impacts per practice is enough to make a meaningful difference for the developing brain.

Other research claimed that wearing soft-shell caps on helmets, implementing Heads Up Football, and using a Riddell helmet with sensors reduced impacts in youth football players over one season, but this study had several issues.[42] First, the Riddell sensor system used in this study is proprietary, so the researchers were not able to say what accelerations qualified a hit as high, medium, or low impact. Given the low overall number of impacts reported, it seems likely that the sensors only triggered with impacts at relatively high accelerations, even for those labeled as low impact. But without knowing what accelerations the players were experiencing, the data can't be compared to other accelerometer studies to suggest these methods improve safety. The only way to show that the Heads Up Football and soft-shell helmets together could actually reduce impacts would be to compare the data to a group that didn't use the interventions. But the study didn't have a comparison group. This study received some media attention claiming that these methods made youth football safer, but that is very misleading. In reality, the study had no data to show the interventions made any improvement in impacts sustained by players. Poor communication from scientists and the media on studies like this can make families think a sport is safer than it is. This is why it is so important to read about research with a critical eye, and never make a decision based on the findings of a single study.

At this point, the jury is still out on Heads Up Football and other similar programs. The decline in practice impacts shown in one study, perhaps due to more dedicated time on low-speed skill training, is encouraging, but it remains unclear how well the skills transfer to full-speed play. The consistent game concussions and impacts across leagues, whether involved in a safety program or not, may back up the claims of former players who don't believe there is such a thing as safe tackling in the full-speed game setting. A linemen incurs hundreds if not thousands of impacts in one season not from tackling but from the blocking that is a regular part of tackle football. They will still incur these impacts no matter what tackling technique is used. And even with "proper" tackling technique, the brain is still moving within the skull.

Helmetless Tackling

Another more drastic idea to improve safety in football has been proposed: remove the helmets altogether. It may seem counterintuitive, but this has roots in the efforts to move to a more rugby-style tackle in football. Helmets can give a false sense of security to athletes, even though their brain is still vulnerable as it moves within the skull.[43] In football, it's thought that players will adopt better hand placement and technical skills in tackling and blocking in part due to the need to better protect themselves without a helmet on.

Limited research has investigated the effect of training without helmets in practice. One study followed high school football players in a helmetless tackling program developed at the University of New Hampshire.[44] This program involves a progression of ten drills performed two to four times per week without helmets or shoulder pads. The drills teach players motor patterns to avoid leading with their head when tackling, and the goal is that they will carry those same motor patterns into helmeted full-contact play. Players in the program experienced around 30 percent fewer impacts in games at time points early and midseason, but the improvements disappeared by the end of the season. Reducing impacts is always a good thing, but it still isn't clear if these helmetless drills can have enough of an effect to substantially reduce overall impacts as well as concussions in youth football. When they put the helmet back on, they may feel protected again and willing to engage in riskier play.

Limited Contact Practice Time

By 2020, over forty states had implemented rules regulating the amount of time a high school football team can spend in full-contact practice, tackling to the ground, and hitting at full speed.[45] Though the amount of time varies by state, the rules usually limit the number of days or minutes per practice or week that can be spent on full-contact play, with some states allowing just fifteen minutes per week in the regular season. The states without any related rules simply allow coaches to decide on the amount of contact their athletes should endure.

In 2014 the Wisconsin Interscholastic Athletic Association passed a rule limiting full-contact practice in high school football to seventy-five minutes in preseason and sixty minutes per week in the regular season.[46] Researchers at the University of Wisconsin–Madison examined the effect of the contact practice limits on concussion rates. Compared to the two seasons before the limits were introduced, the concussion rates overall and in games stayed the same, but the concussion rate in practice dropped by 57 percent with the new rule.

Reducing concussions is an important outcome, but does limited contact time result in fewer impacts? A few early studies suggest the answer may be yes. A youth football team with contact limited to a third of practice time each week had fewer overall impacts in practice compared to two teams without the limitations, though they did experience more impacts in games than the other two teams.[47] Researchers at the University of Michigan studied twenty-six varsity football players from one high school after contact practice time was limited to thirty minutes.[48] The total number of impacts declined an average of 42 percent across all players. It's important to remember that this was only one team. Impact exposure can differ greatly from team to team, owing to coaching style, the culture, and other factors, so research involving more teams will paint a clearer picture. Still, these results are encouraging.

Fewer overall impacts at both the youth and high school levels as a result of reduced full-contact practice time is, no doubt, a great improvement. But we also have to ask ourselves, how many hits are okay? In the Michigan study, the average player sustained 345 impacts and the average lineman 670 impacts over the season after contact practice time was limited.[49] In the youth football study, players on a team with reduced contact still sustained an average of 158 impacts over just fifteen total events, with several players incurring over 200 or even 300 impacts in that time.[50] While these are improvements, players are still experiencing hundreds of impacts over just a few months. Earlier I told you about a study in which former football players saw almost double the risk for having difficulties with executive functions, depression, and apathy when they reached an estimated career threshold of between 1,800 and 2,400 impacts.[51] Using the average numbers of high school and youth impacts from these studies of limited-contact practice time, it would still only take four years of high school play and three years of youth football play to exceed 1,800 impacts. The average lineman would exceed the 2,400 mark with just four years of high school play, not even including impacts from youth football. So, yes, sustaining fewer overall impacts is important, and reduced contact practice time can help. But is it enough? How many impacts are okay for the developing brain, or even the mature brain?

Supporters defending the safety of youth tackle football often argue that they have made more changes to improve safety than any other sport. Sure, they may have made more individual rule changes, but the game still looks pretty similar to what it looked like at the turn of the century. While some changes have had a small positive effect on concussions and subconcussive impacts, other changes have had no effect. Other sports have eliminated the primary source of impacts, but the primary source of impacts, the tackle, is still part of football. More impacts from blocking happen in tackle football as well. Kids are still sustaining hundreds of impacts in a season. We have to keep in mind that *better does not necessarily mean safe*. It's not clear if the changes that have been made to practices make a meaningful difference for the developing brain.

CONCUSSION EDUCATION

The education and awareness surrounding concussions and repetitive subconcussive impacts has grown immensely since the late 2000s. In the United States, every state has passed a concussion law, and the vast majority require concussion education for coaches, parents, or athletes.[52] Some of these laws only apply to the high school level, while others apply to all youth sports.[53] Internationally, concussion education seems to be growing as well.[54]

Unfortunately, more education doesn't necessarily mean more knowledge and better attitudes and behaviors. While a large majority of athletes, parents, and coaches know most symptoms, they often don't know that trouble sleeping, anxiety, nausea, difficulty in school, and being more emotional are symptoms of a concussion.[55] Studies of both athletes and coaches have found that between 13 and 19 percent still believe you have to lose consciousness to have a concussion.[56] While this is a relatively low number, the belief could cause many concussions to go undiagnosed. Education alone is also not enough to cause changes in attitudes and behaviors for many athletes. Once they get on the field, athletes don't want to let their team down by reporting symptoms and having to leave the game. If the game is on the line, athletes are even less likely to report.[57]

Still, awareness of concussions and potential long-term consequences has grown in the twenty-first century. Extensive media coverage and discussion of concussions as well as CTE has occurred worldwide, having both positive and negative outcomes. While this has contributed to increased awareness of the seriousness of these injuries and the need for proper management, it has also led to misconceptions regarding both concussions and CTE. For example, in a survey of more than 1,000 parents, over 55 percent thought that more than one-quarter of athletes would sustain a concussion in high school football each season, and nearly 28 percent thought more than half of all players would sustain a concussion.[58] In reality, the percentage of players who sustain a concussion on a team each season is usually in the single digits. Of course, repetitive subconcussive impacts take a toll, too, and some concussions go undiagnosed, but parents' perception of concussion risk is often far higher than the actual risk.

Whether from the media attention or simply more education bringing more awareness to the injury, the number of concussions diagnosed in sports has increased significantly in the 2010s.[59] Some athletes may be reporting injuries that they didn't realize were concussions before. Others may be reporting their concussions because they now understand how serious the injury can be. Coaches and parents are more aware and may be more likely to notice symptoms in an athlete than before. No matter what the cause, this improved recognition is an important, positive step forward in protecting the brains of our youth athletes.

IMPORTANT CONSIDERATIONS WITH SAFETY-RELATED RULE CHANGES IN YOUTH SPORTS

In many sports, concussions and other serious injuries only happen when something goes wrong: players colliding while diving for a volleyball, a ball to the face in baseball, or a basketball player's head hitting the floor. But in sports like football, rugby, soccer, and hockey, any routine play could cause a concussion or subconcussive impact. Throughout the history of contact sports, changes were made to reduce the incidence of these "freak" injuries and lessen fears of parents, athletes, and fans. [60] When concerns increased, sport organizations and leaders tweaked rules and equipment and claimed that the game was safer than ever. History has repeated itself yet again.

Are youth sports really safer than ever? We have evidence to suggest the answer is yes with youth hockey as a result of the ban on checking at younger ages. However, that is really the only sport with enough evidence to make that claim. Soccer has also eliminated a major source of repetitive impacts and concussions at a young age, but no research has been conducted to tell us whether or not overall impacts or concussions have declined as a result.

While soccer and hockey have made more drastic changes to their game, the idea that the sport of football has been dramatically changed is just untrue. Leagues and organizations have used claims of new techniques, equipment, and education to wrap the sport in a prettier bow, but it is still tackle football. The aspect of the game that is most inherently dangerous is still there. Though tackling techniques are supposedly taught in a "new" way, those techniques are hard to maintain in the chaos of a game. Even if they are effective in reducing impact forces, it may not be enough to make a significant impact on player health in both the short and the long term.

In the debate around the safety of youth sports, there has been a willingness to deny reasonable evidence that makes logical sense in a quest for indisputable proof. The people who are quick to say we don't know everything about CTE or disrupted development from repetitive brain trauma are often the same people who are quick to say that the game is safer than ever, without proof to back up that statement. The changes made in football and some other contact sports may be more like a Band-Aid on a broken leg. It may not be enough to save the players from long-term consequences. Is "safer than ever" safe enough?

Chapter Twelve

Why You Don't Have to Hit at a Young Age to Be a Superstar

I'm not entirely sure that tackling in third grade makes you a better junior in high school. You can play flag football.
—Tony Romo, former NFL quarterback, Dallas Cowboys[1]

There is a myth prevalent in youth sports today. This myth is driven by the $17 billion youth sports industry.[2] It's driven by parents who think it's the only shot their child has to be successful in a sport and by coaches saying it will increase the likelihood that a child will get a college scholarship. It's driven by companies who want parents and teams to purchase their protective equipment. It's the illusion that an athlete has to focus on one sport and play it by the same rules as the older players at a young age to become great at it, get a college scholarship, or go pro. But this is a *myth*. There is no evidence that a child is more likely to have great success at higher levels if they start playing the full-contact version of a sport in elementary school.

In this chapter I will bust the myth that you have to start young and hit young in order to become a great athlete in a given sport. There are many examples of great athletes who didn't start playing their sport until they were in high school. And there are other things a child can do to increase their chances of becoming a great athlete when they are older.

MANY SUPERSTARS DIDN'T PLAY THEIR SPORT AT A YOUNG AGE

There are many star athletes who didn't play the full-contact version of their sport, and in some cases any version of the sport, at a young age. I'll start with football. Some of the greatest players in NFL history didn't play the tackle version of the game until high school. The Concussion Legacy Foundation created an "All-Time Greatest Flag Under 14 Team" to highlight NFL stars who didn't play the game until at least ninth grade.[3] Here are a few examples:

- *Walter Peyton*, the thirteen-year Chicago Bear whom many consider to be the best running back of all time, didn't start playing tackle football until the tenth grade.
- *Lawrence Taylor*, who played thirteen years with the New York Giants and is known as one of the best linebackers of all time, started playing football in eleventh grade.
- *Jerry Rice*, the former San Francisco 49er, often considered the best wide receiver of all time, started playing tackle football in tenth grade. He played twenty seasons in the NFL.
- *Matt Birk*, the offensive lineman who won a Super Bowl with the Baltimore Ravens, started playing tackle football in the tenth grade. He played fourteen seasons in the NFL.
- *Julius Peppers*, the nine-time Pro Bowl defensive end who played seventeen years in the NFL, started playing tackle football in ninth grade.
- *Michael Strahan*, the fifteen-year New York Giant defensive end, didn't start playing tackle football until he was a senior in high school. He grew up in a military family in Germany and worked to develop his fitness and athleticism.[4] He spent his senior year with his uncle in Houston, where he first played football.
- *Warren Sapp*, the thirteen-year NFL veteran and seven-time Pro Bowl defensive tackle, began playing tackle football in tenth grade.
- *Jerome Bettis*, the Pittsburgh Steelers Hall of Fame running back, was an all-city bowler in middle school.[5] He didn't start playing organized tackle football until high school.
- *Tom Brady*, longtime New England Patriots quarterback, seven-time Super Bowl champion, three-time NFL Most Valuable Player, and arguably the best quarterback of all time, played flag football until ninth grade. Would anyone say that Tom Brady's play has suffered

because he didn't start playing the tackle version of the game until high school? Would he be better than the best of all time if he had started earlier?

These are just a few examples of the many great players who waited to tackle until their bodies and brains were more developed. What do they all have in common? They are great *athletes*. You can learn a lot about the game of football and gain athleticism by playing flag football, without the risk of repetitive impacts and other injuries from tackling.

Internationally, there are many examples of rugby stars who didn't play the sport at a young age.[6] Four-time Australian Super Rugby Player of the Year Chris Latham played soccer when he was young. He didn't play his first game of rugby until age eighteen. Tom Court was an Australian university shot put champion before he started playing rugby at age twenty-four. Sixteen months later he made the second national rugby union team of Ireland. Thierry Dusautoir started playing rugby at age sixteen and went on to captain the French national team. In the United States, many rugby national team players didn't play until high school, college, or even after college.[7] Alev Kelter was a rare Division I two-sport athlete, playing both hockey and soccer at the University of Wisconsin–Madison.[8] She started playing rugby after graduating from college. She has since represented the United States in the Olympics and helped the Women's National Rugby Sevens team to its first world championship, gaining MVP honors along the way.

Again, these are just a few examples of successful athletes who started playing their sport in high school or later. And again, the key to their success was their athleticism. They were able to start a new sport and quickly become great at it because they were great overall athletes. Though most players tend to start sports like hockey and soccer young, the aspects of these sports that result in the most repetitive impacts don't have to start at a young age for these athletes to be successful.

In fact, waiting to introduce full-contact play in youth sports could improve the quality of play in contact sports. A focus on skill and athletic ability rather than force in youth could help some players develop more as athletes.[9] Since banning checking before age thirteen in 2011, USA Hockey youth participation has grown substantially, adding over 30,000 new players and countering a decline in athletes from the preceding years.[10] Flag football has grown considerably in recent years too.[11] That growth is introducing more athletes to the game who may stick with it through the high school level.

TACKLING, CHECKING, OR HEADING YOUNG IS NOT THE KEY TO SUCCESS

How likely is it that a youth athlete will get a college scholarship? Despite the beliefs of some parents and athletes, the odds are pretty slim. Most full college scholarships are available at the NCAA Division I level, with very few available through Division II athletics or other college athletic associations. In 2019, 2.9 percent of high school football players went on to play at the Division I level. Only about 1.8 percent earned a scholarship.[12] That equates to a scholarship for less than 1 percent of youth football players. Hockey has the highest likelihood for high school athletes to reach the Division I college level at 4.8 percent of boys and 8.9 percent of girls. About one-quarter to one-third will not receive a scholarship. In soccer, roughly 1.3 percent of male athletes and 2.4 percent of female athletes who played in high school will go on to play for a Division I college, but less than half of those athletes are on scholarship.

The odds of reaching the professional level are far lower.[13] With fewer than two thousand athletes in the NFL and 254 new players drafted each year, only about 1.6 percent of college football players will go pro. That translates to about 0.02 percent of high school players and less than 0.01 percent of youth players. In hockey, 7.4 percent of college players, or 1.8 percent of high school players, will reach the NHL. The odds are just as small or smaller for other sports.

It is incredibly challenging to predict how talented an athlete is by their performance as a child. Among youth Australian football players, prediction of long-term success was poor for athletes who matured at earlier ages.[14] Being better at a sport than peers when a child is young doesn't mean they will stay that way as everyone else matures. Some parents or coaches think that, if a child doesn't seem talented in a sport at a young age, they have little promise. In most cases, this just isn't true. The Australian football coaches thought later-maturing athletes had less long-term potential than early-maturing athletes. Sadly, this led to fewer opportunities and higher dropout rates for later-maturing athletes. Those that stuck with it had to develop other techniques to be successful and, as a result, often outperformed early-maturing athletes later in their careers.

Being great at tackling, heading, or checking as an eight-year-old does not mean that you will be a successful high school player, earn a college scholarship, or go pro. The odds of the latter two are incredibly low in any sport. Introducing contact at an early age doesn't make those odds any better, but it does increase the likelihood of disrupting brain development or even developing a neurodegenerative disease. Even if the risk of developing CTE is very low, is it worth it to subject a child to years of repetitive impacts for a goal they have a 2 percent chance of obtaining, especially when sustaining those impacts doesn't make those chances any higher?

DELAYING CONTACT DOES NOT INCREASE THE RISK OF INJURY

Some people worry that kids who haven't been exposed to tackling, checking, or heading may be at greater risk for injury when they start, especially if they are playing with kids who have already been tackling or checking for several years. What does the science actually tell us?

In hockey, players in most leagues can begin checking when they reach the bantam level, at age thirteen. After the rules delaying checking were put in place, both concussions and overall injuries declined significantly in players under age thirteen. Yet some feared that injury risks would increase at the bantam level, when these athletes started checking, because they had less experience but were bigger and stronger. That was not the case. The majority of studies found either a decrease in injury rates or similar injury rates in bantam-level players with less checking experience.[15] One study actually found lower injury rates in bantam players who were new to checking compared to those who had been checking for two years, and concussions rates were the same between groups.[16] Introducing checking at a younger age has no protective effect, and there are no additional dangers with delaying checking until age thirteen.

Initial evidence suggests that delaying tackling in football does not lead to more injuries either. In a study of high school football players, there was no difference in concussion rates in players who were new to the game compared to those who had been tackling for several years.[17] The inexperienced players had no problem learning contact skills and were at no greater risk of experiencing a concussion in games or contact practices.

Some proponents of youth contact sports have argued that waiting to teach players how to check, tackle, or head the ball will result in them learning bad habits that will increase injuries later. Even if that is a concern, why not just teach good fundamental habits in the first place as a foundation for more advanced skills later? Coaches can emphasize the factors of most concern at the youth level to prepare athletes for play at higher levels.

When it comes to safety, we should be more concerned about that damage that can come from tackling, checking, and heading at young ages. Playing the non-contact version of these sports will ultimately result in fewer career impacts and less overall brain trauma.

KIDS CAN BECOME GREAT PLAYERS IF THEY BECOME GREAT ATHLETES FIRST

Childhood and early adolescence aren't just important times for brain development. They can also be critical times for building overall athleticism. Rapid brain maturation can provide a window of opportunity for developing coordination, motor skills, and motor control that benefit young athletes not only in their sports careers but throughout their lives.[18] This does *not* mean kids should do high-level training or focused sport-specific training. Athletes who specialize in one sport in youth are more likely to get injured, burn out, and drop out of sports at an early age.[19] Neither sport specialization nor high-level training in childhood increase the likelihood that an athlete will be a star. Playing a variety of sports and doing different kinds of physical activity, including free play, is the best way for a child or adolescent to develop athleticism.[20]

Coaches are looking for overall athleticism in their recruits. Former NFL player and University of Michigan football coach Jim Harbaugh has encouraged young athletes to play soccer instead of football until they reach high school.[21] He believes soccer helps young athletes learn important skills such as footwork, coordination, and spatial awareness as well as develop their endurance and conditioning. As he told the *Wall Street Journal*, when evaluating potential recruits, he looks for athleticism in sports or activities outside of football.

IT IS POSSIBLE TO PROTECT THE BRAIN AND BECOME A GREAT ATHLETE

The myth that youth athletes need to endure repetitive impacts to become great in their sport is simply that, a myth. It doesn't even increase the likelihood of making a high school varsity team. Developing athleticism in children is far more important for long-term success than developing sport-specific skills at a young age. You can teach a child to make a tackle, deliver a check, or head a soccer ball when they are older, but skills like agility, spatial awareness, quickness, and complex footwork can be taught young to help kids develop into athletes. Even if a child does not go on to play higher-level organized sports, developing overall athleticism, including flexibility and endurance, sets children up to build fitness and wellness habits into their routines throughout their lives.

Chapter Thirteen

Why the Benefits of Sports Can Be Gained without Repetitive Brain Trauma

Does the psychosocial environment of American football for youth, including parents, coaches, and the sport system, reward massiveness (overweight and obesity, specifically for linemen) in a manner similar to that attributed to the psychosocial environment of gymnastics and figure skating that fosters limited weight gain in girls?
                        —Robert M. Malina, PhD, and colleagues, 2007[1]

As I mentioned in chapter 2, sports can have enormous benefits for kids, including physical and psychological health outcomes, socialization, and learning life skills. These are often cited in the arguments I hear advocating to keep high-contact sports for kids. However, there is absolutely no evidence that says you have to incur repetitive brain trauma in order to gain those benefits. What the research does show is that participating in *any* sport, especially a team sport, can have exceptional positive outcomes for children. This chapter will discuss why the many benefits of sports are not a legitimate argument for allowing children to sustain the repetitive brain trauma that comes with hundreds of impacts in a season.

LIFE SKILLS, SOCIALIZATION, AND PSYCHOLOGICAL
BENEFITS OF SPORTS WITHOUT REPETITIVE IMPACTS

Contact sports like football, hockey, rugby, and lacrosse are team sports that can provide the many great benefits that all sports have to offer. Some say these benefits are a key reason why kids need to tackle, check, or head the ball at a young age. Often this reasoning is aimed at male athletes, arguing that tackling or checking at a young age helps boys develop into young men.[2] They say tackling and checking build positive character traits like doing the right thing, accountability, confidence, self-esteem, learning how to expend maximum effort, facing and overcoming fears, and self-sacrifice for the good of the team. These are all wonderful takeaways from playing a sport. Not one of them requires a child to sustain repetitive brain trauma.

Some supporters of tackle football say the sport is important for building future members of a productive workforce and society. One supporter said that the players carry the work ethic, self-discipline, determination, teamwork, and leadership skills learned on the field into the workforce to "build a better America." Players learn to continually analyze, grow, outsmart opponents, and make quick decisions in pressure situations. Another supporter of tackling said that the violence was an important factor for his success in the business world. (I wonder how many times he has tackled someone in the boardroom!) It's true, the life skills learned in football have value for a career and in life. But these lessons can be learned in other sports and in non-tackle forms of the game too. Violence doesn't have to be part of that. This logic suggests that athletes in high-contact sports are the only people with the skills needed to excel in life. Clearly that isn't the case. There are very successful people who have played sports like football or rugby, and many, many successful people didn't play these, or any, sports.

Athletes can develop lifelong friendships with their teammates, and those relationships can lead to reduced stress, anxiety, and depression as well as better self-image and a sense of belonging with the team.[3] Coaches can become mentors, sharing stories of their own perseverance in difficult times, providing guidance and encouragement for college, and more. These relationships aren't unique to contact sports. The environment fostered by the coach, the team atmosphere, and the attitude carried into it by the athlete have a critical effect on what the athlete gets out of the sport experience. But you don't have to hit your head to make friends or receive mentorship.

Some say the bond of brotherhood is different in sports like football and rugby because, if you mess up, your teammate could get seriously hurt. They argue that this leads to more player accountability and builds stronger bonds with teammates. But reliance on teammates and accountability are key in many other sports, too, including flag football and flag rugby, without the high risk of concussions or repetitive brain trauma. We have to ask ourselves, does an eight-year-old need to play a sport in which they are at risk of serious injury if their teammate screws up? (And you know they will screw up at some point; they're just eight years old.)

I will end this section with an aspect of youth sports that is too often overlooked: they should be *fun*. Every person will probably find some sports more fun than others, but that doesn't mean they can't have fun playing more than one sport. Fun can, and should, be part of any sport. And this seems obvious, but kids don't have to sustain repetitive impacts to have fun.

KIDS DON'T HAVE TO HIT THEIR HEAD REPEATEDLY TO BE TOUGH

I often hear the argument that kids these days are too "soft," and they need to hit each other and experience a little pain to learn to be tough. Toughness involves grit, perseverance, determination, and the drive to push through difficult situations. Kids do need to learn how to get back up when they fall, both literally and metaphorically. Toughness is certainly an important character trait that can be developed and honed through youth sports.

Some people seem to think that toughness can't be learned if you aren't laying your body on the line, smashing into someone on every play. Some conflate toughness with a misconstrued concept of masculinity, believing boys must learn to hit hard and take a hit in order to become men. This antiquated view puts children and their brains at risk. What is the benefit of telling kids that the only way they can show they're tough is to hit another person as hard as they can or to play through a brain injury because they need to sacrifice for the team? While the benefits they gain from sports can help them throughout their life, the damage they can incur from misguided and unnecessary methods to gain toughness could last a lifetime too.

About one million athletes play high school football each year. That represents about 13 percent of all high school-aged boys.[4] Given that girls make up roughly half of the population of high school-aged kids, and less than 1 percent of girls play football, we can estimate that about 93 percent of high school students don't play football. Does this mean that more than 90 percent of the population, including nearly all women, are mentally weak, unable to deal with pain, and lacking grit and perseverance? Of course not.

Actually, I find it quite insulting when people insinuate that tackling, checking, or other impacts from sports are the only way to learn toughness. My parents raised me to be tough. I honed my toughness as a three-sport athlete in non-contact sports. I am not a great runner, and I never thought I would run a marathon. But I did. When my legs were burning by mile fourteen and I had 12.2 miles to go, including big hills, it took some serious mental and physical toughness to continue. These attributes carry over into other aspects of my life. There were times over the three years I was writing this book, while working full-time, that I wanted to quit. But I kept going (obviously, you're reading this). That perseverance to push through and do something hard and out of my comfort zone was developed through my experience in sports. Yet I didn't have to hit my head repeatedly in any of my athletic pursuits to learn that toughness and perseverance. Athletes can develop grit, perseverance, and toughness in any sport, and in many other activities.

REPETITIVE BRAIN TRAUMA, THE BENEFITS OF YOUTH SPORTS, AND CHILDHOOD ADVERSITY

There is a common narrative that sports are a way out of negative circumstances for some kids. Unfortunately, too many kids have to deal with unthinkable tragedy and unimaginable stresses at a young age, like the death or incarceration of a loved one, growing up in a home with substance abuse, experiencing or witnessing violence, experiencing abuse in some form, or living in poverty.[5] As I discussed earlier, exposure to trauma and adversity in childhood can cause physical changes to the brain. Children who experience adversity have been shown to have smaller volumes in the corpus callosum, hippocampus, and amygdala, as well as more activity in their amygdala.[6] The smaller hippocampus volume is associated with having more depression symptoms. Exposure to early life abuse or violence can even accelerate aging and development in the brain. Structures and networks that process fear and emotions, like the amygdala, may mature faster to process what is happening in their environment. Chemicals released in response to stress can cause critical periods to begin early or end early, potentially shortening the amount of time that important structures have to grow.

Participation in youth sports can positively change the brain.[7] But how does repetitive brain trauma through youth contact sports interact with the consequences of childhood adversity? Right now, we don't know. Only one study, with significant limitations, has looked at how participating in middle school and high school sports influenced mental health in young adulthood in those who experienced childhood adversity.[8] Those who stated that they intended to participate in sports when they were in middle or high school were significantly less likely to have been diagnosed with depression or anxiety around fifteen years later. These findings were true for all sports in the study, including football, but no single sport was any more beneficial to mental health in young adulthood than any other. However, this is the only study of its kind.

It's possible that the benefits of playing a team sport provide some protection against the consequences of childhood adversity. It's also possible that repetitive impacts add to the cumulative burden already on the brain from childhood adversity, potentially leading to worse outcomes later in life. Right now, we don't know how all of these factors interact with each other in the developing brain. This is a topic that desperately needs more research.

THE PHYSICAL HEALTH BENEFITS OF SPORTS ARE NOT GAINED BY ALL ATHLETES

We encourage kids to participate in sports, in part, to increase their physical activity and fitness levels. Supporters of tackle rugby for children have argued that delaying tackling will turn young players into "couch potatoes."[9] But removing tackling from the youth level does not remove the running, cutting, jumping, or other physical activity in the sport. It does remove the most dangerous part of the sport for young athletes with rapidly developing brains.

Physical activity levels and the associated fitness benefits can vary greatly from sport to sport. Football is a sport that involves intermittent bursts of activity, and little aerobic endurance activity. On average, players are only on the field in active play for about five to ten minutes of an entire football game.[10] Only 10 percent of football practice time focuses on fitness, while over half of the time is spent on skills.[11] About 37 percent of all practice time is spent sedentary, such as standing on the sideline or in line waiting to do a drill. While male athletes across other sports spend nearly 50 percent of practice time doing vigorous activity, only about 39 percent of football practice reaches that intensity. As a result, football players are unlikely to meet the amount of moderate or vigorous physical activity, nor aerobic activity, necessary to have a significant impact on weight.

For some positions, the bigger you are, the better. An ideal offensive lineman is a large, immovable force. An effective defensive lineman can use his weight and strength to power forward through the offensive line. I have heard the argument that football provides a home for the "big kids," meaning the kids who are overweight and may not be comfortable playing other sports. Some say that football is the only opportunity for these kids to get physical activity. But for kids entering the sport overweight or obese, football may do little to help their weight, and it could even make it worse.

It is common for linemen to be encouraged to gain weight for both their own success and the success of the team.[12] They may feel the need to gain weight to increase their chances of reaching the next level, either college or professional play. If they get there, they may need to gain more weight to compete with their new peers. This weight gain needs to be done in a safe way that emphasizes gaining lean mass rather than fat mass and should be guided by someone with proper training, especially with children and teens.[13] Even athletes who attempt to gain weight in a healthier way, increasing their lean mass, often have to resort to taking in excessive calories to reach or maintain their goal weight. Former All-Pro lineman Joe Thomas told the *New York Times* he ate often and anything he could, including high-fat foods, to gain the weight he needed to play.[14] Weight loss may be frowned upon because of its potential impact on performance, even if for the sake of the health of the athlete.

Weight can be part of football culture, and the largest players are often revered. An average NFL offensive lineman weighed around 250 pounds in the 1970s. In the 2000s, that weight swelled up to an average of 315 pounds.[15] Gilbert Brown played for the Green Bay Packers in the 1990s. This 350-plus-pound defensive lineman (some say he weighed much more) played ten seasons in Green Bay.[16] I remember seeing ads for Burger King's "Gilbertburger," a Double Whopper with extra everything, but hold the pickles. This burger was wildly popular in Wisconsin in 1997. Brown was loved by fans, including kids. As kids do, they try to emulate the stars, in part by eating his burger.

Research has shown a higher prevalence of obesity in football players at the youth and high school levels as well. Before I describe this research, I need to say that much of it uses the athlete's body mass index, or BMI, which is an estimate of a person's amount of body fat. Muscle weighs more than fat, and athletes tend to have more muscle mass. Because BMI is calculated using only height and weight, a person with more muscle mass has a higher BMI, even though they have a lower and healthier body fat percentage. As a result, BMI may overestimate body fat in an athletic person. That being said, the higher the BMI, the greater the likelihood that it accurately represents higher body fat levels.[17]

High school football players are also more likely to be overweight or obese than the general population of boys the same age, including boys in other sports. Around 18 percent of boys ages twelve to eighteen, on average, are overweight.[18] In comparison, research has found that more than one-third of high school football players are overweight, and 14 percent are obese.[19] Around 45 to 55 percent of linemen are overweight or obese, with 9 to 21 percent being morbidly obese. Notably, the BMI of the linemen was not related to the team's success.[20] These athletes being bigger didn't make the team any better.

The situation is similar at the youth level. In one study, boys who played youth football were twice as likely to be obese compared to boys in the average population of the same age, eight to fourteen years old.[21] Forty-five percent of football players were overweight, with 25 percent being obese. If we conservatively estimate that two million youth athletes play football each year, the results of this study would suggest that roughly half a million boys playing youth football in the United States are obese.

While some activity is better than no activity, claiming the tackle form of football is necessary to fight obesity and provide significant physical activity opportunities for children is an overstatement. A sport that glorifies some athletes being overweight and obese is not setting a good example of health and physical activity for kids. Instead, sports should be teaching children healthy lifestyle habits and safe ways to reach a healthy weight that they can carry with them throughout their lives. There is nothing about tackling that makes a young athlete more likely to reach a healthy weight, and for some, it may have the opposite effect.

REPETITIVE BRAIN TRAUMA IS NOT NECESSARY TO GAIN THE BENEFITS OF SPORTS

As adults, many people look back on their time playing competitive sports as one of the best in their lives. Many parents want their kids to have the same wonderful experiences that they did. I know it's hard to imagine life without the sport or sports that helped shape who you are. Basketball, volleyball, and softball played a huge role in my life. I learned many important life lessons through these sports. However, I'm quite aware that I probably would have learned all of those lessons and gained all of the benefits I did had I played soccer or participated in track and field instead. That wasn't my path, and I loved the sports that I did play. But it's likely that my experience could have been just as fulfilling had the sports I loved been different.

In those non-contact sports, I learned grit and the ability to push myself and put in the extra effort it took to win. I learned how to win graciously and, as much as I hated losing, I learned how to lose with class. I learned that, even when I thought I had nothing left, there was always a little more in me. I learned how to set goals and work hard to achieve them. And while learning how to be tough, I was never exposed to repetitive brain trauma.

Sports can provide an avenue for the formation of lifetime friendships and a place where people of many different backgrounds work together toward a common goal. They can give kids a safe and caring community, mentorship from coaches, a place to forget about their hardships for a little while, and many positive skills that help them navigate challenging experiences throughout life. Sports can help children build lifetime physical activity habits. These benefits are some of the many reasons we should not be talking about abolishing any sports for kids. But no benefit from sports is dependent on incurring repetitive impacts. Keeping our contact sports but implementing meaningful changes to minimize, not just reduce, impacts may be the key to helping all children get the greatest lifelong value from being an athlete.

Part IV

The Future of Youth Contact Sports

Chapter Fourteen

How We Can Change Contact Sports to Protect Children's Brains

I'm a firm believer that there's no way that a six-year-old should have a helmet on and learn a tackling drill. . . . Or a seven-year-old or an eight-year-old. They're not ready for it . . . with flag football you can get all the techniques. We'll eventually get to tackling.
—John Madden, Hall of Fame coach and former NFL commentator [1]

Contact sports have a long history deeply ingrained in our culture. Yet change has always been a part of sports. We have adapted our sports in some cases to increase excitement. In other cases, with new knowledge, we have adapted sports to promote the health of athletes.

Changes have been made throughout the history of football. The forward pass was once illegal. When it was first allowed in the 1906 season, many said it would "sissify" the game. [2] Can you imagine football today without quarterbacks? The wedge was eliminated to reduce injuries and improve player safety. The goalposts and hash marks were moved. Spearing was made illegal. [3] More recent changes have been made with the kickoff and penalties for lowering the head to make contact. There are many more examples. For all of these changes, there were concerns at first. Some people said they would ruin the game, but they got used to it and we moved on. The same would happen if tackling was eliminated in youth football today.

Changes have been a part of the history of other sports too. Helmets and face masks were introduced in hockey, and some thought that was a sign of weakness.[4] Now we can't imagine the game without them. Checking was eliminated for young players, and contrary to what the skeptics feared, it helped the game grow.[5] The rule making back passes illegal in soccer in 1992 had many upset, including goalies who now had to use their feet instead of their hands to manage passes back to them from their teammates.[6] Yet this prevented stalling, sped up the game, and increased excitement in the sport. All of our favorite sports have evolved over time.

It's hard to see something we love change, even if it is for the best. If we make changes to the game now that are necessary for the survival of the sport, children years from now won't know the difference; they will just love to play the game. In fact, years from now people will probably look back on the way football and rugby are played today and say they can't believe we let kids tackle. We say the same thing now about how different sports were played in the past.

Now that you know the science behind repetitive brain trauma in youth contact sports and the counters to the bad arguments to maintain the status quo, where do we go from here? Kids are still hitting their heads repeatedly as an inherent part of many sports. This chapter will present realistic changes that could be made to reduce or eliminate the inherent repetitive brain trauma and concussions while maintaining opportunities for kids to play youth sports.

WITHOUT CHANGE, THE FUTURE LOOKS GRIM

Participation in youth tackle football has dropped substantially over the past decade, including more than 17 percent from 2013 to 2017, and that trend continued through the end of the decade.[7] At the high school level, eleven-player football declined by nearly 80,000 players, or 7.3 percent, from 2015 to 2018.[8] Since 2009 the sport has lost players in nearly every state.[9] Even nationally recognized high school football powerhouses, including several in recruiting hotbeds like Texas, Ohio, and Southern California, have not been immune to the decline. Participation in Ohio dropped over 25 percent. Eight- and six-player programs are growing around the country as schools struggle to field eleven-player teams. Other schools have been forced to shut down their programs due to a lack of players and safety concerns.

Fewer players in youth "feeder" systems means there are fewer players being groomed for high school and higher levels of play. The decline in players can make the game more dangerous for those who remain. With fewer substitutes, athletes are playing more downs, in some cases on both offense and defense, leading to even more impacts over a season.

There are several potential reasons for the decline in tackle football participation. Many blame it on sport specialization or the decline in the actual number of high-school-age boys in recent years.[10] Concerns about concussions and repetitive impacts are likely playing a considerable role in the decline. In one survey, 63 percent of people said that tackle football was probably or certainly not safe for kids.[11] Nearly half felt the same way about high school football. Around 40 percent of parents in Arizona said they would not allow their child to play tackle football.[12] In another survey, 85 percent of parents would or might support age restrictions on tackling in football, with 37 percent saying athletes should wait until high school to tackle.[13]

Even NFL stars are starting to question if the repetitive impacts and wear and tear on the body are worth it. In recent years, athletes have retired at younger-than-expected ages, such as Andrew Luck, Chris Borland, and Calvin Johnson, over concerns about their health.[14] The stigma of caring about health being a sign of weakness is slowly starting to fade even at the highest levels of the game, which may lead young players to draw the same conclusions.

Other signs are troubling for the future of football. Leagues at all levels are having a hard time finding companies that will insure them because of concerns about potential costs related to concussions and CTE.[15] Some have suggested that public schools at all levels should not offer football. They argue that it is unethical for institutions to promote education and development of young minds while at the same time offering sports that can have a detrimental effect on the brain.[16] Fewer people are watching NFL games. For example, 12.5 million Super Bowl viewers were lost from 2011 to 2019, which is a 6 percent decline.[17] A person who participates in a sport is more likely to become an avid fan. As a result, a drop in participation in youth leagues can have a downstream effect on elite leagues, media ratings, advertising, and more. Things will need to change if football is going to stay a core part of American sports culture.

Unlike tackle football, participation in flag football has jumped by 38 percent in recent years.[18] Some athletes and their families are making the choice to play this alternative version of football, at least until they are older. Programs all over the country are adding teams as demand for the sport has skyrocketed. There is a hope that the expansion of flag programs will draw children into the game and those kids will continue into tackle football in high school.

Though the decline in football has been greater than in other sports, football is not alone in losing young athletes. Participation in sports overall is down by over two million kids in the last five years.[19] The number of parents in Arizona who are willing to let their children play any contact sport declined by 17 percent from 2017 to 2019, and nearly one-third of athletes said they decided not to participate in a sport because of concerns about concussions.[20] Participation in soccer is also down in recent years,[21] and a survey found that 60 percent of people felt it was probably or certainly not safe for kids to head a soccer ball.[22] The drop in participation is concerning given the many positive outcomes that can come from youth sports, including football. What can be done to maximize brain safety in sports?

ELIMINATE INHERENT REPETITIVE SUBCONCUSSIVE IMPACTS

We will never get rid of all impacts in sports. While the risk is minimal in many sports, people will fall, elbows will accidentally contact heads, and unintended collisions will occur. However, we *can* prevent young athletes from incurring hundreds or even thousands of repetitive subconcussive impacts in a season. Those impacts are *optional*. We may choose to keep them as part of the game for older players, but they don't need to be part of the game for children. We need to continue to adapt our sports at the youth levels to protect their developing brains.

As I have discussed, several sports have already eliminated the primary source of repetitive impacts at the youth level, with bans on checking in hockey and lacrosse and heading in soccer. Injuries in hockey fell substantially after checking was eliminated from the youth game,[23] and participation in the sport has also skyrocketed.[24] Some medical professionals believe hockey could go further to reduce repetitive impacts. The American Academy of Pediatrics recommends that the ban on checking in hockey should be through age fifteen due to the broad physical maturity and size differences of players in the thirteen- to fourteen-year-old bantam age group.[25] Research supports the recommendation. In a 2019 study, bantam leagues without checking saw 56 percent fewer injuries.[26] Delaying the introduction of checking does not increase the risk of injury once players begin checking at older ages.[27] Together this suggests that the health of youth hockey players would benefit if the delayed introduction to checking was extended until age fifteen.

Minimizing Impacts in Football at the High School and Higher Levels

As I discussed in chapter 11, football has made several changes with the goal of improving safety, including increasing education, a focus on tackling technique, and, in some cases, reduced contact practice time. Of course, "safe" tackling technique may be forgotten in the heat of a game. This combination of changes may help to some degree to improve the safety at the high school and higher levels, but more can be done.

Abolishing the three-point stance could greatly reduce repetitive brain trauma for linemen. Most linemen start every play with one hand on the ground, head down, then explode forward off the line, often colliding with each other helmet first. By starting in an upright athletic position rather than in the three-point stance, one study found linemen could experience 40 percent fewer head impacts.[28] Pop Warner youth football was the first organization to eliminate the three-point stance in 2019.[29] Leagues at all levels of play should follow suit.

The sport could also go further to eliminate, or nearly eliminate, repetitive impacts in practice. Many states have limited full-contact practice time, but in most cases, this could be taken even further. Removing or substantially limiting tackling in practice to only a few times per year or fifteen minutes per week at most does not reduce the quality of game play. There are many examples of teams that have largely removed tackling or hard contact from practice and been very successful. The American Heritage School in Plantation, Florida, has removed tackling from nearly all practices, tackling in no more than four practices per year.[30] The non-contact practices have more than prepared them for game play. They have won four Florida state championships in recent years. Ramapo High School in New Jersey followed a similar model, not tackling each other to the ground at all over the season.[31] They won a state title in 2018.

Dartmouth hasn't tackled players to the ground in practice since 2009. Yet they finished at or near the top of the Ivy League standings for most of the 2010s, including two Ivy League championships.[32]

Dartmouth coach Buddy Teevens and his staff analyzed tackling for the most effective technique to reduce missed tackles, and they focus on those details when practicing with robotic tackling dummies. They cut their missed tackles in games by two-thirds, despite never tackling each other in practice. Coach John Gagliardi of St. John's University eliminated tackling and hard contact from practice in the 1950s.[33] He led his team to forty-four winning seasons, twenty-seven conference championships, and four national championships over his coaching career. All of this goes to show that you don't have to hit hard in practice to win games. Instead, eliminating tackling in practice can keep players healthy and ready for game day.

Some have argued that the lack of practice tackling will lead to more injuries in games. However, a study of high school football players found that concussions in games remained the same as previous years after contact practice was limited to sixty minutes per week.[34] This early evidence indicates that players can to learn to tackle without regularly tackling each other in practice and without raising the risk of concussions in games. In fact, it could lead to fewer game concussions. Athletes who sustain concussions often tend to have more impacts in the day or week leading up to the injury, suggesting that eliminating impacts during the week in practice might reduce concussions in games.[35] Time, and future research, will tell.

Eliminating tackling in practices costs little to no money and takes few if any resources. Players can practice technique by approaching and wrapping up other players without taking them to the ground. For little money, coaches can get creative with things like mattresses to create tackling dummies. It costs the team nothing, not money or quality of play, to eliminate repetitive impacts in practice and benefit the health of players.

Eliminate Repetitive Impacts from Tackling in Youth Football

While reducing contact practice might be enough at older levels, we have to ask ourselves if it is okay for the rapidly developing brain of a child to sustain any repetitive brain trauma inherent to a sport. As you have read, repetitive impacts can have negative consequences for the developing brain. The only way to eliminate repetitive brain trauma in youth football is to eliminate tackling. We can't eliminate every accidental impact, but we can eliminate those that we know happen as part of every routine tackle football play.

Non-tackle options like flag, TackleBar, or flex football can be great ways to introduce the game of football to kids without repetitive impacts that can affect the brain. In flag football, play ends by pulling a flag from a belt around the athlete's waist. Flex football includes blocking, but no head or shoulder contact or tackling.[36] The ball is called down by two-hand touch. Flex football is promoted as a high-speed environment where athletes can learn the physical game without repetitive impacts. TackleBar football is played nearly the same way as tackle football, with the same pads and helmets.[37] Each player wears a harness with two foam bars on their back. Instead of tackling, the "tackler" is taught to wrap their arms around the ballcarrier and rip at least one bar from their back. One study found that injury rates were lower in TackleBar compared to tackle football, and it could be a great bridge between flag and tackle.

In these non-tackle forms of football, kids can develop and sharpen important skills like throwing, catching, and footwork. Coaches can teach the rules of the game, and players can learn how to run plays. Non-tackle football could get more kids interested in the game, and those kids may love it and want to play tackle football as they get older. Tackling technique could be gradually introduced through skills camps or limited only to minimal impacts through controlled practice drills, similar to soccer heading, until the age that full-contact play begins.

The Concussion Legacy Foundation is promoting "Flag Football Under 14," or essentially non-tackle football before high school.[38] This would allow even later-maturing athletes to get through a peak time of brain development before being exposed to repetitive brain trauma. Delaying tackling not only gives the brain more time to develop without disruption, but it also decreases the total number of impacts they will incur over their career. Playing a non-tackle form of football until high school doesn't mean that the quality of play will suffer at higher levels, either. For example, the youth football program in Middlebury, Vermont, has been a flag program for years, and their high school program has been one of the best in the state for a decade.[39] Many successful players waited to tackle until high school, and you can learn nearly all football skills without sustaining hundreds of impacts. So why not wait?

As with reducing contact in practice, some have argued that games could be more dangerous when children are older if they don't learn to tackle when they are young. There is absolutely no evidence to support this. In one study, high school football players with less prior experience had no greater risk of sustaining a concussion compared to those with more prior experience.[40] This was on teams in a state where contact practice was limited to just sixty minutes per week, but the less experienced players were still able to learn to tackle without an increased injury risk. Supporting evidence also comes from hockey. When players reached the bantam level at age thirteen, those who had played in a league without checking at the peewee level had the same injury and concussion rates as those who had played in a peewee league that allowed checking. Delaying contact does not make the game more dangerous at older levels.

Puberty is less a factor if tackling is delayed until high school, or at least late middle school. Later-maturing athletes would have more time to meet the physical levels of their early-maturing peers before they start tackling. Players would have more time to develop athleticism and motor control. Young children often don't have the motor skills and coordination to master the complex motor requirements of tackling. As players get older, stronger, and more athletic, they have the motor control necessary to effectively learn so-called proper tackling skills.

Many NFL greats spanning decades of play have come out in support of flag football before high school, including tight end Zach Ertz, wide receiver Jordy Nelson, linebacker DeAndre Levy, NFL coach Mike Ditka, and Hall of Fame coach and NFL commentator John Madden.[41] Quarterbacks Tony Romo, Jim McMahon, Kurt Warner, Ben Roethlisberger, and Brett Favre have also voiced support for flag football for youth athletes. Drew Brees, who played flag football until high school, cofounded Football 'N' America, a non-contact youth coed football league that is open to students in kindergarten through tenth grade.[42]

While the American Academy of Pediatrics agrees that hockey should delay checking until age fifteen, they refuse to take a similar stand on tackling in football.[43] Yet they concede that "repetitive trauma has no clear benefit." It is unclear why they support banning the act that causes the most injuries and concussions in one sport but not in another.[44] Unfortunately, this medical group that should be providing guidance for parents is only adding to confusion.

As of 2020, six states have introduced legislation attempting to ban tackle football before a certain age: Illinois, Maryland, California, New York, New Jersey, and Massachusetts.[45] While several have failed, other bills are still under review. This change won't likely be driven by youth leagues without government intervention. Bans on checking and heading happened, in part, because hockey, lacrosse, and soccer have a single national governing body (USA Hockey, US Lacrosse, and US Youth Soccer). Nearly all leagues and teams, and in some cases players, are registered with their sport's national organization. With one governing body overseeing nearly all programs in the country, they could implement these changes in the best interest of the athlete without worrying about competition from other groups willing to allow these behaviors.

In youth football, USA Football and Pop Warner football are both popular nationwide organizations that sponsor youth football leagues, and other independent leagues exist as well. Leagues fear that dropping tackle football will cause them to lose players and money. If USA Football decided to offer only flag football before middle school or high school, a Pop Warner league could swoop in and offer a new tackle football league. Even if it's in the best interest of young athletes, these organizations won't likely make a significant change like this on their own.

Some parents say that they wouldn't let their child play tackle football anyway, but they want it to be their decision, not a government mandate. While that is understandable, there are many laws that protect children's safety when parents or other adults might not, even though they might be acting with the best of intentions. For example, if we didn't have laws for infants using car seats, how many parents would hold their baby on a car ride? Maybe the child is sick, and they want to comfort her. Maybe the child cries when he's in the car seat and it's just a short trip. Maybe they want to feed the baby without pausing the trip. There are many reasonable motivations why a parent might make that decision. The odds are low that anything bad will happen, right? But what if an accident did happen? The law is there to keep the child safe.

I want to emphasize that a ban on tackling for young players is *not* a ban on football. It is a ban on tackling. They use the same type of ball. There is still a line of scrimmage and a battle for field position. Touchdowns are worth the same number of points. Players still pass and run the ball. The difference is that plays don't end with a tackle. A child is not pulled to the ground, linemen aren't running into each other the same way on every play, and head impacts aren't an inherent part of the game. All of the good that comes from the sport can happen without tackling and repetitive impacts. It is still football even if kids aren't tackling.

Other countries are having similar debates about tackling. A ban on contact before age twelve has been called for in Australian football.[46] In England, rugby players can typically start tackling at age eight, and some feel that is far too young.[47] Removing tackling from these sports at young ages would, like in football, reduce repetitive impacts and protect the maturing brain.

While we will never eliminate every single impact in sports, *repetitive* hits to the head are optional. We should be taking every step possible to eliminate unnecessary head impacts that are inherent to different youth sports. Soccer has survived without heading at the youth levels. Hockey and lacrosse have survived without checking at youth levels. Football, rugby, and Australian football could eliminate tackling at the younger ages and survive that change too.

ENFORCE RULES TO PROTECT PLAYERS

Officials can play an important role in creating a safe culture on the field, court, or ice. Most sports have rules banning dangerous contact. When officials enforce rules, players are less likely to play in an overly aggressive or dangerous way.[48] High school football players surveyed knew that helmet-first tackles could result in a penalty and potentially an ejection from the game, but they did it anyway, likely because they didn't believe the rule would be enforced.[49] In rugby, illegal tackles, such as high tackles, are far more likely to result in injuries.[50] Officials need to enforce rules banning these tackles, and the penalties need to be sufficient to discourage athletes from using these tackle techniques anyway. If players know the rules aren't being enforced, why would they bother following them?

I once had a mother tell me that she let her son play tackle football because she was concerned about the direction that flag football was heading as her son got older. The players had become more aggressive, diving for flags and running into each other. Over time, she felt like they were tackling anyway, and she was more comfortable if her son was wearing a helmet and pads. I can completely understand this concern. While I support flag football at younger ages, rules need to be enforced. Injuries in flag football happen most often in out-of-control plays and poorly regulated practices. Players should stay on their feet, and illegal contact should be strictly penalized.

Enforcing rules extends beyond games. States and youth organizations often provide very little oversight to ensure rules outlawing specific drills or limiting contact practice time are being followed. Some coaches go above and beyond to ensure they follow these rules. Other coaches feel that they can get away with ignoring these rules, so they do.[51] Increased oversight to hold coaches accountable is critical to the safety of kids playing contact sports.

Rule enforcement is also needed at the highest levels of all sports so that kids don't normalize these behaviors. For example, the NFL should enforce rules designed to discourage leading with the head and enforce greater penalties on those who do, such as an automatic one-game suspension. These infractions will happen less if the penalty is more severe. If kids watch their idols make these plays on Sundays, many will want to play like that in their own games.

EFFECTIVE CONCUSSION EDUCATION AND INFORMED CONSENT

All athletes and parents should be well informed of the potential risks of a sport before they agree to participate. Parents and athletes often sign consent forms, but it doesn't mean that they actually know the risks.[52] There are no guidelines on what is required for informed consent with concussions and repetitive impacts in sports. Ideally, the process should include written *and* in-person education. Young athletes can't consent to play on their own, but they should be informed of the risks and involved in the process. If the duty to become informed is solely placed on the parent or athlete, it is easy for the leagues or organizations to claim that they have no liability, even if they don't provide all relevant information. Parents and athletes can only give *informed* consent if they are actually informed.[53]

While concussions aren't the only concern, they are serious injuries that must be identified and managed correctly. To improve reporting by athletes, concussion education and the culture of sports go hand in hand. Education will not be effective if the culture that considers leaving the game a sign of weakness persists. Yet we cannot change the culture without effective education that focuses on changing attitudes and behaviors. Education focusing on the potential short- and long-term consequences of not reporting may have a greater positive effect on attitudes and beliefs about reporting.[54] The culture shift away from the warrior mentality and effective concussion education need to include not only the individuals involved but also the system of sports as a whole.[55] Athletes, coaches, parents, officials, teammates, fans, teachers, schools, sports organizations, and community members all interact, and their attitudes and behaviors influence each other. They all play a critical role in creating the culture that promotes the health of athletes above all else.

Concussion education is not "one size fits all." It needs to be tailored to the audience based on the sport and the individual or group's role in the sport. Officials are in a prime position to notice concussed athletes on the field or ice, but they need to know what to look for. Medical providers must stay up to date with the best practices for concussion diagnosis and management. Concussion education for athletes should be specific to the sport and include steps for what to do if they suspect that their teammate has a concussion. If teammates encourage reporting and support these athletes, more concussions may be reported.

Many young athletes receive information about concussions from their parents. Concussion education should teach parents what signs and symptoms to look for in their child, how to overcome barriers to reporting, how to seek care, potential consequences, and potential benefits that come from reporting the concussion.[56] It should also provide guidance for how to talk with their child about concussions. If the parents know what a concussion is but don't know how to discuss it with their child, the education may not be effective.

Most athletes want coaches to be engaged in concussion education because they want to know where their coach stands on the issue.[57] In one study, just 10 percent of coaches discussed concussions with their players before the season.[58] Athletes may perceive this as a sign that reporting is discouraged. The coach should be explicit with their team about their feelings on safety and the value of reporting concussions. Coach concussion education should include tips for talking about the injury with their athletes and encouraging a safe reporting environment. Coach education also needs to be low cost and accessible. Coaches from areas with lower average incomes often do not receive the education that coaches from higher income areas do.[59]

We should not assume that athletes are always deliberately hiding concussions based on rational decision making. The intention to report may be there in most cases, but in an important game, that rational thinking can be lost with the roar of the crowd and the intensity of the situation. Rational thinking may also be impaired by the concussion itself. A child may not understand their injury, and we can't give them the entire burden to report. Coaches, teammates, officials, parents, and medical providers can play a crucial role by noticing potential signs of a concussion and removing the athlete from play or encouraging them to report their symptoms.

Several steps can be taken to improve concussion education in sports:

A Clear Definition: Given the many misconceptions still held about the injury, it is crucial that concussion education provides a clear and thorough concussion definition. Research has found that athletes at all levels of play report more previous concussions when they are given a definition of what a concussion is.[60] Education should provide all potential symptoms, including having a "ding," seeing stars, or having their bell rung. We can't expect athletes at any age to give an accurate concussion history or report new injuries unless they know that what they're feeling is actually a concussion.

Reporting Skill: One goal of concussion education should be to enhance reporting skill, which is the understanding of how to report or knowing how to learn how to report a concussion in a variety of situations. In a study from the University of Wisconsin–Madison, athletes with better reporting skill had better intentions to report their concussion.[61]

Educate Early and Often: Concussion education often only happens at the beginning of the season and then is forgotten about as the season moves on.[62] Coaches and athletic trainers can give their teams regular reminders of key points about reporting, and parents can talk to their children about concussions throughout the season.

Start Young and Make It Age Appropriate: Children learn attitudes toward injuries early in their sport experience, and age-appropriate concussion education has to start before negative attitudes about reporting concussions become ingrained.[63] Children should be given tangible examples set in the sports they are playing. High school athletes need education delivered with the understanding that teens are more prone to risk-taking behaviors. Many youth and high school athletes aren't familiar with medical language, and they need the concussion-related terms put in words and phrases they can understand.

Get Creative with Concussion Education: As a professor, I know that standing up in front of my classroom and lecturing for an hour is not the best way for my students to learn. The same goes for concussion education. Athletes aren't likely to be engaged in the process or learn very much if they are just given a piece of paper with some symptoms on it or sit through a lecture about it. A combination of methods, including videos, games, discussions, and interactive demonstrations, will be far more effective. If they learn about concussions in a fast-paced gamelike setting, they may be more apt to remember what to do when a concussion happens in the same setting. Parents can incorporate such education while playing catch outside or watching a game on TV. Getting athletes involved and engaged is one key factor in making the information stick.

IMPROVING THE CULTURE OF SPORTS

Improving the safety of youth sports in the community involves not only the rules of the sport itself but also the culture and attitudes surrounding the sport. The culture of sport can become part of our identity, and changing that culture can feel like changing part of ourselves. I grew up watching football, but it's hard for me to watch the game now. I've seen how the trauma sustained in the culture of the sport can give its heroes a brain disease that can take their mind, their work, their family, and eventually their life. It's also hard for me *not* to watch football because it's something that I have enjoyed for so much of my life. It feels a bit like a part of me is missing on Saturdays and Sundays in the fall. I want to feel good about watching again, and there are many others out there who feel the same way I do. But the culture needs to change.

Professional leagues should lead by example. Athletes can set an example by reporting concussions and encouraging youth in the sport to do the same. Illegal impacts should be denounced by all involved. Instead, coaches, players, and fans often voice their anger and yell at officials. Kids see that and think the officials are just being unfair and those hits are okay. In hockey, the NHL is in denial that the game can put some players at risk of long-term brain damage.[64] The league will not condemn fighting, though it adds nothing to the game but injuries. It's not part of international play, and those games are great entertainment. Most importantly, they are setting an example for younger athletes who see the pros fight and think it is a normal part of the game.[65] Support from the highest levels of all sports is crucial for promoting a culture of safety at younger levels.

Youth and high school coaches, leagues, and organizations should work to counter the culture that requires aggression to prove dedication to the team. Removing checking at the youth level has both reduced injuries and shifted the culture of aggression. When hockey players start checking, coaches should devote time to promoting the intent of separating the puck from the opposing player rather than inflicting a bruising hit.[66] When football or rugby players start tackling, coaches should emphasize wrapping up the athlete, not inflicting a big impact on the opponent. Coaches who promote unsafe play, such as encouraging dangerous contact drills, extending contact time in practice beyond allowed limits, encouraging aggression, or demeaning players for reporting concussions, should be held accountable.[67]

Fair-play leagues in hockey have helped to change the culture. Teams receive points for having minimal penalties, and those points factor, along with wins and losses, in their league standings at the end of the season.[68] Therefore, teams who minimize aggression are rewarded, and the focus remains on speed and skill in games rather than force. Other sports could create similar leagues that discourage illegal and harmful play and encourage a culture of safety.

There is a difference between being an assertive, aggressive player and playing with aggression. An aggressive player is willing to play hard at all times to help the team while maintaining sportsmanship. Aggression carries more risk of harm to themselves or other players. Athletes who play with more aggression tend to sustain more impacts and may be more likely to injure another player. Coaches should recognize players with higher aggression and take steps to intervene to maintain the safety of all their players.

Mental toughness is, at least in part, a learned skill that can be shaped in childhood and adolescence. If a parent or coach is constantly criticizing a kid's skills or the play of the team, young athletes may only see criticism as a negative and may never understand the value of constrictive criticism.[69] On the flip side, setting too low of expectations and avoiding situations that require athletes to show grit and perseverance won't develop mental toughness either. Fostering a culture of toughness that is measured with ample support and promotion of safety can create an environment in which a young athlete can thrive athletically and personally. Like many things in life, it's all about balance.

Some people believe kids aren't playing certain sports because they just don't want to work hard. Many kids have the grit and determination needed for success, but some channel that into a sport or activity that carries fewer risks. The transformation from "boy to man" is happening in different venues, but it's still happening. Not wanting to develop a brain disease or have a concussion disrupt school and social life, and not wanting to inflict that possibility on other humans, doesn't mean an athlete is soft or lacking in character. Parents not wanting that for their kids aren't just helicopter parents. Valuing health is not weakness.

MEANINGFUL CHANGE CAN HELP SAVE YOUTH SPORTS

No sport comes without risk. Concussions and head impacts will happen, but they are far more common in some sports than others. It's true that flag or other non-tackle forms of football still carry a risk of injury, but well-structured practices and rule enforcement may minimize that risk. Still, eliminating the repetitive subconcussive impacts at the youth level will go a long way to protect the brains of our youth athletes.

Everyone involved in sports, including athletes, parents, coaches, leagues, schools, medical providers, fans, and other stakeholders, need to take an active role in helping the culture and play of youth sports evolve. There is fear that some sports will look different in the future, at least at the youth levels. It's true, they might look a little different. But they look different today than they did a century ago, and they are still great sports. Rule changes and culture shifts for the sake of safety won't ruin the game. They will allow the game to survive and evolve in a way that improves safety for youth and, hopefully, draws more kids to play sports.

Chapter Fifteen

What Families and Athletes Can Do to Stay Safe in Youth Sports

If the current debate about concussions is to yield a safer outcome for kids than more than a century of similar conversations has, it must involve a much deeper acknowledgment of what researchers—and, really, everyone else—have already known for decades: Repeated collisions are not safe for human bodies or brains.
—Kathleen Bachynski, PhD, assistant professor of public health, Muhlenberg College[1]

The choice of whether or not a child should play a sport isn't always easy. Many factors can sway a young athlete and their family one way or another, including community pressure, availability of other sports, socioeconomic status, a child's desire to play, and so much more. Both the parent and the child might lose their own social circle if the child doesn't play a sport. The decision of if and when it is right for each child to start playing a sport that has a higher risk of injury to both the brain and the body can be a difficult one. And if families decide to let their child play a full-contact sport, what do they need to do to keep young athletes safe?

Although this chapter is geared toward families with young athletes, it has important information for coaches and others who are committed to keeping young athletes safe. I will discuss important considerations when deciding whether or not to play a sport, as well as key steps to take to ensure a child is playing in the safest environment possible, no matter what sport they are playing.

CONSIDERATIONS IN THE DECISION TO PLAY A SPORT

There are many factors families need to consider when deciding whether or not a child should play a given sport, especially when the sport has a high risk for concussions or repetitive subconcussive brain trauma. Here are a few things to consider:

Focus on the Best Interest of the Child

Many parents want their children to have the same great experiences that helped shape them into the people they are. I absolutely understand that, and I would want the same for my child. But ultimately, parents need to be able to push those feelings aside to act in the best interest of their child. It is hard to be objective when certain sports are so ingrained in our personal story and our culture. Families have to think about what is best for the child over the love of a specific sport.

I've heard some people say that just a few years of youth play isn't that bad for the brain. As you have read, repetitive impacts in youth can potentially interfere with brain development. Aside from that, the risk of getting CTE probably is very low with just a few years of youth contact-sport play. But there is no guarantee the child will only play for a few years. What if they love it and they are talented? It's unlikely that a child would want to give it up, which means more cumulative years and more cumulative head impacts. By simply delaying the start of tackling, checking, or heading, they will experience fewer lifetime impacts.

A Child Is Not Capable of Making This Decision by Themselves

Some children really want to play a certain sport, like football. Families want their child to be happy, so they let them play. But this argument implies that a child's brain is capable of weighing the pros and cons, which simply isn't the case. Child and adolescent brains aren't developed enough to fully understand the potential short- and long-term risks of playing sports with a high risk of repetitive brain trauma and truly make an informed decision.

The parts of the brain involved in processing emotions mature before the parts of the brain involved in reasoning, judgment, and decision making. Children and teens are focused on the present. The fear of missing out can greatly influence their choices. They want to play a sport with their friends, and they will focus on that short-term outcome. Even if they know that there could be long-term consequences, it is hard for them to understand what that would really mean for their lives. Can a ten-year-old fully understand what life could be like in their forties, fifties, or sixties because they hit their head a lot as a child? Of course not. It's even harder for a child to comprehend the risks when they have parents, coaches, and others in the community pressuring them to choose the team over their own health. Whether the child ultimately ends up playing a contact sport or not, they shouldn't be the only ones in charge of making that decision.

Some families are afraid to keep their child out of something that they want to do. But the truth is, parents make decisions kids don't like every day because it is in the child's best interest. Parents limit the amount of soda and candy their child consumes or how much screen time they have. Many parents make their child wear a bike helmet. If a parent decides not to let their child play a sport because they want to protect their brain, it would be just another decision they make for their child's health, even though the child may not like it or understand it at the time.

Talk to a Child about the Decision to Play a Sport

Although parents or caregivers need to be the primary decision makers, kids should be involved in the conversation. Parents should talk about the science in simple terms with concrete examples, and the child should be encouraged to ask questions along the way. Parents should be honest that they don't know all of the risks but they care about the child's brain, now and when they grow up. The child might decide they want to protect their brain too. This can also show kids how to advocate for their health, and it may empower them to do the same in the future.

Let the child know that playing sports is a great thing, but their brain is important. They can try a variety of other sports, build their athleticism, and maybe transition into the sport of interest when they are older. It's also important to sympathize with the pressures they may be feeling from other kids and discuss ways to deal with those pressures. This is not a one-and-done conversation. It's something that needs to be revisited season to season.

Make Sure Kids Are Still Involved in Sports or Other Physical Activity

Physical activity and team interaction can have so many great benefits. If your child doesn't play one sport out of concern for their health, make sure their health is still benefiting from playing another sport or participating in some form of regular physical activity. Although all sports carry some risks, the risks are higher in some sports than others. Deciding not to play a high-risk sport only to choose another high-risk sport might not be the best answer. Yet leaving a sport altogether may not be the best option either. Playing a non-contact or limited-contact version of a high-risk sport may be a great compromise.

It's also crucial to make sure kids aren't quitting a high-risk sport to focus on only one sport. At least eleven medical and health organizations have advised against specializing in one sport at least in childhood if not through high school.[2] Contrary to popular belief, specializing early does not increase a kid's chances of success, getting a scholarship, or going pro. It does increase the chances that they will burn out early or develop an overuse injury and quit at a young age.[3] Giving a child the chance to play multiple sports will help them find sports that they really enjoy and want to play not only as a kid but also throughout their lives.

RESPECT A FAMILY'S DECISION NOT TO HAVE THEIR CHILD PLAY

If you decide to let your child play a contact sport at any level, that is your decision for *your* child. A friend of mine has a thirteen-year-old son who is a very talented athlete. When he was younger, she discussed the potential consequences of playing youth tackle football with her husband and son. Together they decided that flag football was the best choice for him, which he excelled at. This was the right decision for her family and her son. Then came the pressure from all angles. The child's friends at school pressured him to play tackle football. Other parents pressured his parents as well, saying that the team needed their son. This was particularly hard for the boy's father, who was getting pressure from other dads.

This is wrong. No one should pressure other parents to let their children play a certain sport. Think about the message being sent, that a sixth-grade football team is more important than a child's health. What if he had a heart condition that may not cause any problems but came with a very small risk of a heart attack if he raised his heart rate too high? If the family decided it was not a risk worth taking, would other parents question that? If the team wasn't doing well, would they say, "But the risk is so low, why don't you let him play?" Of course not. Yet some people don't think about the potential risks of repetitive brain trauma this way, likely because consequences may not show until years later. Yes, these risks might be low, but they are real. Is the potential success of the team more important than the future health of someone else's child? Does a coach or another parent have the right to make that decision about someone else's child when that decision could impact their long-term health and cognitive function? The answer is a resounding *no*. Parents should also talk to their children about the importance of respecting the decision of another family and not putting pressure on their friends.

If you are a parent receiving this pressure, stand your ground. If you choose not to let your child play a sport because of legitimate concerns about safety, you are not in the wrong. Don't let others pressure you into a decision you are not comfortable with. You are the one concerned with the best interest of your child and their future, while the priorities of others are likely far from that. Your child is the one who has to live with any consequences.

WHAT FAMILIES SHOULD DO WHEN THEIR CHILD PLAYS A SPORT

There are several things to keep in mind when a child starts playing a sport. They apply to all sports, but some are even more important when it comes to sports with a high risk of concussions or repetitive subconcussive brain trauma. Parents should take these steps any time their child starts a new sport or at the beginning of a new season with a new coach.

Get to Know the Coaches

Whether the child is playing a contact or a non-contact sport at the youth or the high school level, parents should be comfortable with the coaching staff and confident that coaches do all they can to keep their players safe. Injuries will happen in any sport, but coaches can choose drills and create a culture on the team that can help limit serious injuries. Talk to other parents about the culture the coach fosters on the team. A coach who fosters a negative culture, whether that is demeaning players or disregarding safety, is not a coach a child should be playing for. There are many great coaches out there who are wonderful mentors and role models for athletes. These coaches use positive coaching and constructive methods to encourage athletes.

Find out if all coaches have had proper training not just on concussions but also on other safety issues like heat exposure and CPR. The coach-to-athlete ratio should be low enough that coaches can interact with each athlete and maintain safety in all drills. Ensure the coach follows safety rules, such as limiting contact time in practice or avoiding certain drills. Ideally football and rugby coaches will choose not to have athletes tackle to the ground often or at all.

It's okay to watch part of practice at the beginning of the season. This is not permission to be *that* parent, the one who harasses coaches or tells them what to do. Remember, youth coaches are often volunteers, and they usually have the best of intentions. However, it's permission to observe the environment a coach creates and the way they run their practices. It is okay to kindly ask the coach about their training, coaching style, and motivation methods. If you aren't comfortable with what you see and hear, it's okay to choose not to have your child play on that team.

Make Sure Equipment Fits Correctly

Though equipment will never fully prevent concussions, the equipment that is worn must fit properly. All brands and types of helmets need to fit correctly to protect against catastrophic injuries. Football helmets should fit snugly around the head without gaps between the cheek and face.[4] The head should be covered from a point two finger widths above the eyes to the base of the skull. The chin strap should be tight, and the ear holes should align with the ear canal. The helmet should not slide or move easily on the head, and the face mask should not get in the way of the player's vision. Helmets and headgear in any sport should fit based on the manufacturer guidelines.

Educate Yourself

Though most sports programs provide some concussion education, it is often limited. Go above and beyond that and learn more. You are already off to a good start reading this book. The CDC also has helpful resources for parents.[5] Concussions can happen in any sport or other activities, like playing in the backyard with friends. Kids spend the most time around their family, and family members should know how to recognize if a child might have a concussion and what to do if they suspect a concussion.

Talk to Your Child about Brain Trauma in Sports

Parents play an important role in educating kids about concussions and repetitive impacts in sports. This should be a topic of discussion at the beginning of the season, with reminders sprinkled throughout the season. The conversation should be age appropriate and include scenarios that the child will understand when talking about what a concussion is, how to report it, and who to report it to. For example, if a player is injured in a game on TV, parents can talk to their child about what they could do in that situation in their own game. Children and early adolescents tend to be more concrete thinkers, and they may not understand why they need to follow certain steps after their injury in order to play their sport again.[6] Keep reinforcing the importance of reporting concussion symptoms for their health and their performance in sports.

Some parents are concerned that they will instill fear into their child by having these conversations. But the same could be said for telling a child that they need to wear a bike helmet or their seatbelt. If it is handled in a fearful way, then it might instill fear. But if that conversation is rooted in the benefits of sports and the benefits of health for the brain, it doesn't have to be fearful at all. They should do their best to play as safely as possible and minimize impacts for both their sake and the sake of the kids they are playing with. And they should tell an adult if they don't feel right after an impact.

WHAT TO DO IF YOU SUSPECT A CHILD MIGHT HAVE A CONCUSSION

A child with a concussion may not be able to explain what they are feeling. A parent or caregiver knows their child's normal mannerisms and behaviors. If something seems off, that's probably because it is. If you are concerned they may have a concussion, ask them to explain how they feel, in their own words. A child's report of their symptoms often doesn't match a parent's report initially after a concussion. Parents may miss symptoms that the child hasn't thought to tell them about. You can find a symptom list on the CDC website mentioned in note 5 above. Ask about those symptoms in words they will understand. The more you know about what they are experiencing, the better you and their health care provider can monitor their symptoms and progress them back into academics, sports, and life.

It's important to seek help from a health care provider who has up-to-date training in concussions. Simply being a doctor doesn't mean a person knows how to manage the injury. Research has shown that many physicians have at least some gaps in concussion knowledge or don't use recommended guidelines for managing the injury.[7] They may be excellent health care providers, and some are very knowledgeable about concussions. However, concussion knowledge and best practices are rapidly evolving, and it can be hard to keep up when they have so much to know about many aspects of medicine. We ask so much of primary care and emergency health care providers. We can't expect them all to be experts on everything. Athletic trainers spend more time in their professional training learning about concussions and often manage these injuries more frequently than most physicians. Though not all athletic trainers have up-to-date training either, many are very knowledgeable about concussions.

If you aren't sure if the clinician has up-to-date concussion education, it's okay to ask. If a clinician is upset that you are asking about their qualifications and training with regard to the injury, that's probably not someone you want caring for your child anyway. Concussion clinics that specialize in the injury may be a great option if you have one in your area. (Of course, it is important to check with insurance carriers to see if they cover those clinics.)

ADVOCATING FOR HEALTH CAN BE A SKILL LEARNED THROUGH SPORTS

Parents play a critical role in advocating for the health of their children. By educating themselves and having important discussions with their children about brain safety in sports, they can create a culture in their home that both values sports and values health. External pressures from coaches and others in the community can make this advocacy mentally and emotionally challenging. However, parents can use this experience to teach their children how to stand up for themselves, withstand peer pressure, and advocate for their own health. This can be just another way that sports can teach children important life skills.

Chapter Sixteen

What You Can Do to Improve the Safety of Youth Sports in Your Community

The most important thing for parents is establishing an element of fun and imagination. I think that's really key.
—Kobe Bryant, eighteen-time NBA All-Star [1]

Protecting and supporting brain health in youth sports involves many community-level factors. Teachers and school staff can help concussed student-athletes return to learning. Athletic trainers provide medical care for youth athletes. Organizations that offer youth sports can provide non-contact or limited-contact sports for children. Most importantly, all stakeholders play a role in ensuring that sports stay fun for kids to play. This chapter will discuss what you can do in your community to ensure both safety and opportunity for all kids in youth sports.

ENSURE ALL KIDS HAVE ACCESS TO SAFE SPORTS

All children should have the opportunity not only to play sports but to play sports that don't involve repetitive subconcussive brain trauma. Unfortunately, several factors are keeping more and more kids out of sports today. As youth sports becomes more commercialized, many kids are being priced out of participation. [2] Middle- or high-income families that live in larger communities often have more options to choose sports that are safer for their children. Those that live in smaller rural areas or low-income communities may not have those same options or enough kids to form leagues for some sports.

You can play a role in creating opportunities for children to play non-tackle sports in your community. Talk to other parents about creating flag football or touch rugby programs, for example. You could help to create leagues in different non-contact sports too. If there isn't enough support or there aren't enough players, try working with nearby towns or neighborhoods to start a league. It's so important for children to have affordable and safe opportunities to obtain the many benefits of sports.

ADVOCATE FOR ATHLETIC TRAINERS IN YOUTH SPORTS

Athletic trainers are medical providers for physically active people, and you will commonly find them in the sports setting. They don't help people lift weights. They are well educated on the medical recognition and care of injuries that can come from physical activity, including the proper recognition and management of concussions. In fact, athletic trainers in sports settings often manage concussions on a regular basis. Compared to athletes with little or no access to athletic trainers, athletes who attend high schools at which athletic trainers are regularly available are more likely to have their concussions diagnosed and to undergo the medically recommended return-to-play protocol.[3]

Leagues should also ensure that athletic trainers are available to provide medical care at youth sporting events. It can be hard for coaches to determine if an eight-year-old has a concussion or if they just forgot a play because they're eight years old. Many coaches appreciate having athletic trainers on the sidelines. They can take the burden off of coaches and ensure that concussions are diagnosed in youth athletes. But when the athletic trainer is only at games, the player may not receive proper follow-up care. If the athletic trainer is regularly available to the team, concussed athletes are more likely to go through the appropriate return-to-play protocol. You can advocate and fundraise to have athletic trainers on the sidelines of youth games, and even at practices, in your community. You may be able to partner with a local hospital or clinic or hire an athletic trainer for per diem work.

ENSURE YOUR LOCAL LEAGUES HAVE CONCUSSION EDUCATION AND MANDATORY PROTOCOLS

All youth leagues, schools, and sports organizations should provide concussion education and have a protocol describing what to do if they suspect an athlete may have a concussion. It should include a concussion definition with all possible signs and symptoms and instruct coaches, officials, or parents who suspect an athlete has a concussion to remove the athlete from play and seek care from a qualified medical provider. You can encourage your school or sports organization to create a protocol that is in line with current medical recommendations.

ADVOCATE FOR CONCUSSION TRAINING FOR EDUCATORS AND SCHOOL STAFF

Learning and schoolwork can worsen concussion symptoms. It is critical for school districts to develop a "return to learn" policy for concussed students and ensure all educators and staff understand how to help students with concussions. Educators with no concussion training may not believe the student-athlete has an injury that they can't see. Teachers and school staff with concussion training may be better prepared to provide academic accommodations that will keep concussed athletes learning on pace without worsening their symptoms.

Communication is key. Families should communicate with teachers about the athlete's injury and limitations. Teachers should keep open communication with families to discuss their progress and any setbacks with symptoms. Communication between teachers and athletes is also key to putting the athlete at ease in an already stressful situation.

The goal in returning to school is to help the athlete learn without making their symptoms worse. The concussed athlete should rest their brain for at least a day after the injury. However, prolonged cognitive rest can actually worsen symptoms. Within a few days the student-athlete can slowly begin school activity for short periods of time. They can gradually increase academic activities, modified at first, and then moving toward normal activity, as long as no activity aggravates symptoms.[4] You can advocate for concussion training for all educators and staff and the creation of a "return to learn" policy in your local school or district.

MAKE SPORTS FUN

The pressure and culture created by parents, coaches, and other adults has been blamed as one reason why the average child stops enjoying a sport and drops out by age eleven.[5] If playing a sport isn't fun, they are less likely to stick with it. Having fun doesn't mean kids aren't striving to do their best and learning toughness, grit, perseverance, and other lessons along the way. Yes, winning is more fun than losing, but that isn't the primary concern for most kids. With good coaching and the right support, children can thrive in sports and be happy while doing it.

We also should not be recruiting kids for college based on how they play in fifth or sixth grade. Yes, some kids that age already have recruiting pages online. Talent prediction is poor for young kids. When they hit puberty, a lot can change. Think about what it can do to a child to have so much hype around them only to have others mature and catch up. The pressure to succeed would be immense, and it can be devastating to them if they don't meet or exceed the expectations adults put on them at such a young age. Is it fair for adults to set such high expectations and put so much pressure on a child based on their abilities as a ten-year-old?

Physical activity shouldn't feel like a chore. It should be something that they enjoy. Of course, it may not be enjoyable all of the time. Conditioning is part of sports and often a part that athletes would say is their least favorite. But keeping conditioning and sport activities age appropriate is key.[6] What is appropriate for a teenager may not be right for a child. Training that is too physically or emotionally intense can lead to injury or burnout, and neither are fun for the young athlete. Kids also need rest. They should do a different activity at least two or three days each week instead of playing their sport. This variety and time away from a sport allows recovery, reduces the risk of overuse injury, and keeps sports fun. Overall, they should enjoy the sport, despite the tough parts. The benefits of sports aren't seen if children drop out early.

BE AN ADVOCATE FOR CHANGE IN YOUR COMMUNITY

When fighting for change, focusing on what can be gained or maintained can be more influential than what would be lost. For example, focusing on how the benefits of sports can occur in a non-contact version of football and how many successful athletes played flag football may be more effective than focusing on the elimination of tackling. Discussing a reduction in repetitive brain trauma may not convince those fighting to keep these sports as they are, but discussing the potential benefits for the brain and body, including fewer injuries that would keep a child out of the sport, could potentially carry more sway.[7]

You have the power to advocate for brain safety in youth sports as well as proper concussion management in your community. You can create opportunities for children from all backgrounds to play sports without the risk of repetitive subconcussive impacts. In the process, you can set a great example for children of how they, too, can get involved and make positive changes in their community in their future.

Conclusion

How Much Do We Have to Know and How Bad Do the Risks Have to Be?

> But while I applaud that concern for impacts to the head is now acknowledged more widely, I'm conscious that many still prioritise the "look of the game" over player safety, lamenting that the game has become "dull" or "soft" since it was "cleaned up."
> —Alan Pearce, PhD, associate professor, La Trobe University [1]

The "show me the data" standard has been used by industries for nearly a century to claim that something should be proven unsafe before it is regulated or changed. [2] Companies claimed there was no definitive proof that leaded gas was a health hazard, so it shouldn't be banned because it benefited consumers. Tobacco companies denied the dangers of smoking. In a 2018 *Revisionist History* podcast, Malcolm Gladwell gives the example of miners' asthma, the breathing issues that coal miners suffered from after working in the mines. [3] Coal companies denied the dangers and even went so far as to say it was protective because the miners had a slightly lower prevalence of tuberculosis, a claim that was based on poor and biased research. Gladwell asks, "What level of proof do we need about the harmfulness of some activity before we act?"

Data is never perfect, and every study has limitations. Even a topic with a wealth of data supporting one side will have a few studies with contradicting findings. Industries use such contradictions to create uncertainty and claim scientists are overreacting. But the public health burden should not be on scientists to prove something is unsafe. It should be on the industry to prove it *is* safe.

Sports organizations have taken a similar road. When a study comes out that supports their stance, they promote it without acknowledging the limitations of the research. Yet, when a study comes out that goes against the organization's interests, they focus only on the limitations as a way to discredit it. This creates uncertainty in the eyes of parents and athletes alike, encouraging them to conform to community and social standards that could be putting young athletes at risk of both short- and long-term consequences.

We have known for decades that contact sports carry danger for athletes, but the risks were largely ignored. When former athletes in sports like football, rugby, and hockey have spoken out about the consequences of brain injuries, some fans have said they knew what they were getting into. Yet CTE was only diagnosed in athletes in these sports in the twenty-first century. Most former players didn't know the true risks. For current players, leagues are still minimizing the risks and making claims that the game is safer than ever. Saying that athletes know what they're getting into and it's an easy choice simply allows fans to feel better about celebrating brutality for the sake of entertainment.

At the youth level, medical and educational organizations in the 1950s said football was "no game for boys to play."[4] Yet here we are, continuing to have this conversation. Some campaigns are fighting to "protect the game" and show parents it is safe. They should be more concerned about protecting the developing brains of young players than the act of tackling. The American Academy of Pediatrics, which stood against youth tackle football in the 1950s, has not supported a ban on tackling in youth football today. Yet they are willing to support a ban on checking in youth hockey until age fifteen. Inaction or inadequate action can have consequences.[5] But what is the harm in delaying the age a child starts sustaining repetitive impacts in any sport?

Common sense tells us that hitting our heads is bad for the brain. If repetitive brain trauma occurred in the classroom, on a field trip, or even in gym class, parents would be irate. Why is it okay on the field, ice, or pitch? The fact that these sports are so ingrained in our culture and our lives makes it hard to change them, even for the sake of safety.

There is precedent for promoting caution and change without definitive proof. In public health, we must make decisions based on the best available evidence, despite uncertainty, while we are waiting for more definitive proof. When people, especially children, could be harmed in the meantime, we have to act on what we know now.

Though we don't understand every aspect of the long-term consequences of repetitive concussive and subconcussive brain trauma, there is growing evidence to suggest that these impacts are bad for our brain, especially when they happen in childhood and adolescence. We have a lot to learn, but we know enough now to warrant eliminating repetitive impacts at the youth level and limiting those impacts as much as possible at older levels. Banning certain sports as a whole or deciding not to let a child play sports in general due to the potential risks takes away critical opportunities for kids to be physically active, improve mental health, make friendships, learn life lessons, and more. If we make meaningful changes now, millions of innocent kids can play sports without repetitive impacts while we wait for definitive answers.

I've seen what CTE can do to a person. I've seen the fear in the eyes of former athletes of all ages who are concerned their symptoms are from repetitive impacts in sports and are fearful of what their future holds. I've heard the stories of desperation from families who don't know how to help their loved ones. I don't want that to happen to any child who just wants to play a sport they love with their friends.

Acknowledgments

I am tremendously grateful for the endless encouragement and support of so many wonderful people. First and foremost, to my family. My husband, Brian, has been my rock throughout this roller coaster of a process. He has encouraged me through every step, read and reread every chapter, helped with the bibliography, made countless dinners while I was writing, and made me laugh when I needed it most. He supports my dreams unconditionally, and I am so blessed to have his love and constant encouragement.

I am so grateful to my parents for their encouragement and for always reminding me that I am capable of great things. And a special thank you to my mom for reviewing every chapter. She proofread and gave feedback on my papers in middle school and high school, and she was still up to the task years later for this . . . slightly larger project. Thank you, Mom!

I am incredibly thankful to Dr. Margene Anderson for reading and giving comments on my chapters, for helping me with my "field research," for hours of conversation on this topic, and for sharing her perspective and experiences. Most importantly, I am thankful for our friendship.

I don't know how I would have made it to this point without the help of Jennie Nash. I am so grateful for her willingness to take me on and guide me through the proposal process. Her positivity, enthusiasm, and spirit made a stressful process exciting and achievable. Thank you so much to Joëlle Delbourgo for her guidance and support. Thank you to Suzanne, Deni, Jehanne, and everyone at Rowman & Littlefield who brought this book into the world.

I am so appreciative of the continued mentorship and support of Dr. Robert Stern. Thank you to Chris Borland for the inspiring conversation and encouragement of this project. Thank you to Drs. Robert Cantu and Chris Nowinski for their support of this project. The research and advocacy contributions made by these men to the field of brain trauma in youth sports are beyond measure.

Thank you to all of my research collaborators, including my lifelong friends from the CTE Center and everyone at the Psychiatry Neuroimaging Laboratory (especially Marty and Inga). Thank you to all scientists studying this important topic, and all people advocating for safety in sports. This is important work, and you are valued. And to all of the athletes and families that have participated in the studies described in this book, thank you for helping to move this science forward.

I am blessed to have incredible colleagues at the University of Wisconsin–Madison. Thank you to Dr. Pat Hills-Meyer for our conversations on the topic, for your feedback on parts of the book, and most importantly for your support and understanding throughout this process. Thanks to all of my friends and colleagues in the Department of Kinesiology for your support and encouragement.

Thank you to my wonderful family for your love and encouragement. To my friends TL, Dale, Ali, Matt, Jon, Noelle, Eric, Lauren, Ellen, Sean, and all those I didn't name, your kind words and encouragement helped me get here. TL, thank you for your amazing friendship and for being so understanding throughout this process. I promise I will say yes more now that this is all done.

Notes

1. WHY WE SHOULD CARE ABOUT REPETITIVE BRAIN TRAUMA IN YOUTH SPORTS

1. Bill Simmons and Kevin Clark, "The Future of Football with Chris Borland," *Ringer NFL Show*, December 28, 2017, https://www.theringer.com/2017/12/28/16803842/future-of-football-with-chris-borland.

2. "Hardest Pop Warner Hit Ever," YouTube, November 7, 2009, https://www.youtube.com/watch?v=JRvBqwHJo8Q.

3. Bryan R. Cobb et al., "Head Impact Exposure in Youth Football: Elementary School Ages 9–12 Years and the Effect of Practice Structure," *Annals of Biomedical Engineering* 41, no. 12 (2013): 2463–73, https://doi.org/10.1007/s10439-013-0867-6.

4. USA Hockey, "Hockey in the United States: A Growing Game," November 8, 2018, https://www.usahockey.com/news_article/show/966542.

5. Hockey Canada, "Annual Report July 2016–June 2017," http://cdn.hockeycanada.ca/hockey-canada/Corporate/About/Downloads/2016-17-annual-report-e.pdf.

6. International Ice Hockey Federation, "Survey of Players," https://www.iihf.com/en/static/5324/survey-of-players, accessed May 24, 2020.

7. FIFA.com, "FIFA Survey: Approximately 250 Million Footballers Worldwide," April 3, 2001, https://www.fifa.com/who-we-are/news/fifa-survey-approximately-250-million-footballers-worldwide-88048.

8. Sports and Fitness Industry Association, "Soccer Participation in the United States," June 14, 2018, https://medium.com/@sfia/soccer-participation-in-the-united-states-92f8393f6469.

9. USA Rugby, "Record Breaking Numbers Mark Special Year for Global Game," July 10, 2019, https://www.usa.rugby/2019/07/record-breaking-numbers-mark-special-year-for-global-game/.

10. Aspen Institute, "2019 State of Play: Trends and Developments in Youth Sports," https://assets.aspeninstitute.org/content/uploads/2019/10/2019_SOP_National_Final.pdf.

178   *Notes*

11. NCAA, "Estimated Probability of Competing in College Athletics," http://www.ncaa.org/about/resources/research/estimated-probability-competing-college-athletics, accessed April 16, 2020.

12. NCAA, "Estimated Probability."

13. Christopher Nowinski, "Youth Tackle Football Will Be Considered Unthinkable 50 Years from Now," *Vox*, April 3, 2019, https://www.vox.com/2019/3/27/18174368/football-concussion-brain-injury-cte-youth-football.

14. Pop Warner, "Ages and Weights," https://www.popwarner.com/Default.aspx?tabid=1476162, accessed May 24, 2020.

15. Jesse Mez et al., "Clinicopathological Evaluation of Chronic Traumatic Encephalopathy in Players of American Football," *JAMA* 318, no. 4 (2017): 360–70, https://doi.org/10.1001/jama.2017.8334.

16. Sameer K. Deshpande et al., "Association of Playing High School Football with Cognition and Mental Health Later in Life," *JAMA Neurology* 74, no. 8 (2017): 909–18, https://doi.org/10.1001/jamaneurol.2017.1317.

17. Ken Belson, "To Allay Fears, N.F.L. Huddles with Mothers," *New York Times*, January 28, 2015, https://www.nytimes.com/2015/01/29/sports/football/nfl-tries-to-reassure-mothers-as-polls-and-studies-rattle-them.html?login=email&auth=login-email.

2. HOW YOUTH SPORTS CAN PROVIDE A LIFETIME OF BENEFITS

1. "Study: On Average Child Quits Sports at Age 11," *ESPN*, August 2, 2019, https://www.espn.com/espn/story/_/id/27308702/study-average-child-quits-sports-age-11.

2. Julian Ayer et al., "Lifetime Risk: Childhood Obesity and Cardiovascular Risk," *European Heart Journal* 36 (2015): 1371–76, https://doi.org/10.1093/eurheartj/ehv089; Seema Kumar and Aaron S. Kelly, "Review of Childhood Obesity: From Epidemiology, Etiology, and Comorbidities to Clinical Assessment and Treatment," *Mayo Clinic Proceedings* 92, no. 2 (2017): 251–65, https://doi.org/10.1016/j.mayocp.2016.09.017.

3. A. Llewellyn et al., "Childhood Obesity as a Predictor of Morbidity in Adulthood: A Systematic Review and Meta-Analysis," *World Obesity* 17 (2016): 56–67, https://doi.org/10.1111/obr.12316; Ayer et al., "Lifetime Risk."

4. Kerli Mooses and Merike Kull, "The Participation in Organised Sport Doubles the Odds of Meeting Physical Activity Recommendations in 7–12-Year-Old Children," *European Journal of Sport Science* 5 (2019): 1–7, https://doi.org/10.1080/17461391.2019.1645887.

5. Centers for Disease Control and Prevention, "Physical Activity Guidelines for Americans," 2nd ed., 2018, https://health.gov/sites/default/files/2019-09/Physical_Activity_Guidelines_2nd_edition.pdf.

6. Data Resource Center for Child & Adolescent Health, "National Survey of Children's Health," 2018, https://www.childhealthdata.org/browse/survey/results?q=6854&r=1.

7. Stewart A. Vella and Dylan P. Cliff, "Organised Sports Participation and Adiposity among a Cohort of Adolescents over a Two Year Period," *PLOS ONE* 13, no. 12 (2018): e0206500, https://doi.org/10.1371/journal.pone.0206500.

8. Desiree Leek et al., "Physical Activity during Youth Sports Practices," *Archives of Pediatrics & Adolescent Medicine* 165, no. 4 (2019): 294–99, https://doi.org/10.1001/archpediatrics.2010.252; Eric E. Wickel and Joey C. Eisenmann, "Contribution of

Youth Sport to Total Daily Physical Activity among 6- to 12-Yr-Old Boys," *Medicine & Science in Sports & Exercise* 39, no. 9 (2007): 1493–1500, https://doi.org/10.1249/mss.0b013e318093f56a.

9. Leek et al., "Physical Activity"; Keith M. Drake et al., "Influence of Sports, Physical Education, and Active Commuting to School on Adolescent Weight Status," *Pediatrics* 130, no. 2 (2012): e296–304, https://doi.org/10.1542/peds.2011-2898.

10. Chloe Bedard, Steven Hanna, and John Cairney, "A Longitudinal Study of Sport Participation and Perceived Social Competence in Youth," *Journal of Adolescent Health* 66, no. 3 (2019): 352–59, https://doi.org/10.1016/j.jadohealth.2019.09.017; Rochelle M. Eime et al., "A Systematic Review of the Psychological and Social Benefits of Participation in Sport for Children and Adolescents: Informing Development of a Conceptual Model of Health through Sport," *International Journal of Behavioral Nutrition and Physical Activity* 10, no. 98 (2013): 1–21, https://doi.org/10.1186/1479-5868-10-98; Martin Camiré and Pierre Trudel, "Using High School Football to Promote Life Skills and Student Engagement: Perspectives from Canadian Coaches and Students," *World Journal of Education* 3, no. 3 (2013): 40–51, https://doi.org/10.5430/wje.v3n3p40.

11. Lisa S. Gorham et al., "Involvement in Sports, Hippocampal Volume, and Depressive Symptoms in Children," *Biological Psychiatry: Cognitive Neuroscience and Neuroimaging* 4, no. 5 (2019): 484–92, https://doi.org/10.1016/j.bpsc.2019.01.011.

12. Bedard, Hanna, and Cairney, "Longitudinal Study of Sport Participation."

13. Emily Pluhar et al., "Team Sport Athletes May Be Less Likely to Suffer Anxiety or Depression Than Individual Sport Athletes," *Journal of Sports Science and Medicine* 18 (2019): 490–96.

14. Gorham et al., "Involvement in Sports."

15. Johannes W. de Greeff et al., "Effects of Physical Activity on Executive Functions, Attention and Academic Performance in Preadolescent Children: A Meta-Analysis," *Journal of Science and Medicine in Sport* 21, no. 5 (2018): 501–7, https://doi.org/10.1016/j.jsams.2017.09.595; Nils Opel et al., "White Matter Microstructure Mediates the Association between Physical Fitness and Cognition in Healthy, Young Adults," *Scientific Reports* 9, no. 1 (2019): 12885, https://doi.org/10.1038/s41598-019-49301-y.

16. Joseph E. Donnelly and Kate Lambourne, "Classroom-Based Physical Activity, Cognition, and Academic Achievement," *Preventive Medicine* 52 (2011): S36–42, https://doi.org/10.1016/j.ypmed.2011.01.021.

17. Camiré and Trudel, "Using High School Football to Promote Life Skills."

18. Katrijn Opstoel et al., "Personal and Social Development in Physical Education and Sports: A Review Study," *European Physical Education Review* 26, no. 4 (2020): 797–813, https://doi.org/10.1177/1356336X19882054.

19. Lee Smith et al., "Association between Participation in Outdoor Play and Sport at 10 Years Old with Physical Activity in Adulthood," *Preventive Medicine* 74 (2015): 31–35, https://doi.org/10.1016/j.ypmed.2015.02.004.

20. Centers for Disease Control and Prevention, "Physical Activity Guidelines."

21. Traci R. Snedden et al., "Sport and Physical Activity Level Impacts Health-Related Quality of Life among Collegiate Students," *American Journal of Health Promotion* 33, no. 5 (2019): 675–82, https://doi.org/10.1177/0890117118817715.

22. Kevin M. Kniffin, Brian Wansink, and Mitsuru Shimizu, "Sports at Work: Anticipated and Persistent Correlates of Participation in High School Athletics," *Journal of Leadership & Organizational Studies* 22, no. 2 (2015): 217–30, https://doi.org/10.1177/1548051814538099.

23. USA Hockey, "Hockey in the United States."

3. WHY SPORTS CULTURE NEEDS
A TRANSFORMATION

1. William R. Thayer, "Topics from the President's Report," in *The Harvard Graduates' Magazine*, 14th ed. (Boston: Harvard Graduates' Magazine Association, 1906), 406.

2. "Bandura and Bobo," Association for Psychological Science, May 18, 2012, https://www.psychologicalscience.org/publications/observer/obsonline/bandura-and-bobo.html.

3. Jason P. Mihalik et al., "Effect of Infraction Type on Head Impact Severity in Youth Ice Hockey," *Medicine & Science in Sports & Exercise* 42, no. 8 (2010): 1431–38, https://doi.org/10.1249/MSS.0b013e3181d2521a.

4. Steven R. Corman et al., "Socioecological Influences on Concussion Reporting by NCAA Division 1 Athletes in High-Risk Sports," *PLOS ONE* 14, no. 5 (2019): e0215424, https://doi.org/10.1371/journal.pone.0215424.

5. Tiffany M. Bisbey et al., "Safety Culture: An Integration of Existing Models and a Framework for Understanding Its Development," *Human Factors* (2019): 1–23, https://doi.org/10.1177/0018720819868878.

6. Andrew M. Kuriyama, Austin S. Nakatsuka, and Loren G. Yamamoto, "High School Football Players Use Their Helmets to Tackle Other Players Despite Knowing the Risks," *Hawai'i Journal of Medicine & Public Health* 76, no. 3 (2017): 77–81.

7. Ben Shpigel, "Luke Kuechly Joins N.F.L.'s Under-30 Retirees Club," *New York Times*, January 15, 2020, https://www.nytimes.com/2020/01/15/sports/football/luke-kuechly-concussions-retire.html?auth=login-email&login=email.

8. Dan Pontefract, "Bob Costas versus NBC, the NFL and the Question of Values," *Forbes*, February 19, 2019, https://www.forbes.com/sites/danpontefract/2019/02/19/bob-costas-versus-nbc-the-nfl-and-the-question-of-values/#147d88b01024.

9. Alison Lukan, "Evolution of the Goalie Mask: NHL Goaltending Equipment Has Come a Long Way," NHL.com, February 21, 2017, https://www.nhl.com/bluejackets/news/evolution-of-the-hockey-goalie-mask/c-286870424.

10. Thomas A. Daniel et al., "North American Football Fans Show Neurofunctional Differences in Response to Violence: Implications for Public Health and Policy," *Frontiers in Public Health* 6, no. July (2018): 1–9, https://doi.org/10.3389/fpubh.2018.00177.

11. Rory Taylor, "Andrew Luck Gets to Walk Away. Not All Athletes Can," *Talk Poverty*, August 30, 2019, https://talkpoverty.org/2019/08/30/andrew-lucks-gets-walk-away-not-athletes-can/.

12. Julie M. Stamm et al., "Awareness of Concussion Education Requirements, Management Plans, and Knowledge in High School and Club Sport Coaches," *Journal of Athletic Training* 55, no. 10 (2020): 1054–61, https://doi.org/10.4085/1062-6050-0394-19.

13. N. Cook and T. N. Hunt, "Factors Influencing Concussion Reporting Intention in Adolescent Athletes," *Journal of Sport Rehabilitation* 29, no. 7 (2020): 1019–23, https://doi.org/10.1123/jsr.2019-0419; Zachary Y. Kerr et al., "Motivations Associated with Non-disclosure of Self-Reported Concussions in Former Collegiate Athletes," *American Journal of Sports Medicine* 44, no. 1 (2016): 220–25, https://doi.org/10.1177/0363546515612082.

14. Christine M. Baugh et al., "Frequency of Head-Impact–Related Outcomes by Position in NCAA Division I Collegiate Football Players," Journal of Neurotrauma 32, no. 5 (2015): 314-426, https://doi.org/10.1089/neu.2014.3582.

15. Corman et al., "Socioecological Influences"; Kerr et al., "Motivations Associated with Non-disclosure"; Emily Kroshus et al., "Concussion Under-Reporting and Pressure from Coaches, Teammates, Fans, and Parents," *Social Science and Medicine* 134 (2015): 66–75, https://doi.org/10.1016/j.socscimed.2015.04.011.

16. Kyle Winters, "NCSA: Are Athletic Scholarships Guaranteed for Four Years?," *USA Today*, July 23, 2019, https://usatodayhss.com/2019/ncsa-are-athletic-scholarships-guaranteed-for-four-years.

17. Kelly Sarmiento, Zoe Donnell, and Rosanne Hoffman, "A Scooping Review to Address the Culture of Concussion in Youth and High School Sports," *School Health* 87, no. 10 (2017): 790–804, https://doi.org/10.1111/josh.12552.

18. Cook and Hunt, "Factors Influencing Concussion Reporting."

19. Kroshus et al., "Concussion Under-Reporting."

20. Kerr et al., "Motivations Associated with Non-disclosure"; Jessica Wallace, Tracey Covassin, and Erica Beidler, "Sex Differences in High School Athletes' Knowledge of Sport-Related Concussion Symptoms and Reporting Behaviors," *Journal of Athletic Training* 52, no. 7 (2017): 682–88, https://doi.org/10.4085/1062-6050-52.3.06.

21. Emily Kroshus et al., "Concussion Reporting, Sex, and Conformity to Traditional Gender Norms in Young Adults," *Journal of Adolescence* 54 (2017): 110–19, https://doi.org/10.1016/j.adolescence.2016.11.002.

22. Aaron J. Zynda et al., "Continued Play following Sport-Related Concussion in United States Youth Soccer," *International Journal of Exercise Science* 13, no. 6 (2020): 87–100.

23. Johna K. Register-Mihalik et al., "Demographic, Parental, and Personal Factors and Youth Athletes' Concussion-Related Knowledge and Beliefs," *Journal of Athletic Training* 53, no. 8 (2018): 768–75, https://doi.org/10.4085/1062-6050-223-17.

24. R. Kyle Martin et al., "Concussions in Community-Level Rugby: Risk, Knowledge, and Attitudes," *Sports Health* 9, no. 4 (2017): 312–17, https://doi.org/10.1177/1941738117695777.

25. Barrow Neurological Institute, "Barrow Concussion Survey: Fewer Parents Let Kids Play Contact Sports," August 22, 2019, https://www.barrowneuro.org/press-releases/barrow-concussion-survey-fewer-parents-let-kids-play-contact-sports/; Sarmiento, Donnell, and Hoffman, "Scooping Review."

26. Rebecca Cover, Trevor Roiger, and Mary Beth Zwart, "The Lived Experiences of Retired Collegiate Athletes with a History of 1 or More Concussions," *Journal of Athletic Training* 53, no. 7 (2018): 646–56, https://doi.org/10.4085/1062-6050-338-17.

27. Christine M. Baugh et al., "Perceived Coach Support and Concussion Differences between Freshmen and Non-freshmen College Football Players," *Journal of Law, Medicine, and Ethics* 42, no. 3 (2014): 314–22, https://doi.org/10.1111/jlme.12148.

28. Sarmiento, Donnell, and Hoffman, "Scooping Review."

29. Wallace, Covassin, and Beidler, "Sex Differences."

30. Rebecca D. Boneau, Brian K. Richardson, and Joseph McGlynn, "'We Are a Football Family': Making Sense of Parents' Decisions to Allow Their Children to Play Tackle Football," *Communication & Sport* 8, no. 1 (2018): 26–49, https://doi.org/10.1177/2167479518816104.

31. Philip E. Kearney and James See, "Misunderstandings of Concussion within a Youth Rugby Population," *Journal of Science and Medicine in Sport* 20, no. 11 (2017): 981–85, https://doi.org/10.1016/j.jsams.2017.04.019.

32. Emily Kroshus et al., "Threat, Pressure, and Communication about Concussion Safety: Implications for Parent Concussion Education," *Health Education & Behavior* 45, no. 2 (2017): 254–61, https://doi.org/10.1177/1090198117715669; Register-Mihalik et al., "Demographic, Parental, and Personal Factors."

33. Boneau, Richardson, and McGlynn, "'We Are a Football Family.'"

4. WHY KIDS REALLY DO HIT THAT HARD

1. Nowinski, "Youth Tackle Football."
2. Jaclyn B. Caccese and Thomas W. Kaminski, "Minimizing Head Acceleration in Soccer: A Review of the Literature," *Sports Medicine* 46 (2016): 1591–1604, https://doi.org/10.1007/s40279-016-0544-7.
3. Kathryn L. O'Connor et al., "Head-Impact–Measurement Devices: A Systematic Review," *Journal of Athletic Training* 52, no. 3 (2017): 206–27, https://doi.org/10.4085/1062-6050.52.2.05.
4. O'Connor et al. "Head-Impact–Measurement Devices."
5. Logan E. Miller et al., "An Envelope of Linear and Rotational Head Motion during Everyday Activities," *Biomechanics and Modeling in Mechanobiology* 19, no. 3 (2019): 1003–14, https://doi.org/10.1007/s10237-019-01267-6.
6. O'Connor et al., "Head-Impact–Measurement Devices."
7. Eamon T. Campolettano et al., "Development of a Concussion Risk Function for a Youth Population Using Head Linear and Rotational Acceleration," *Annals of Biomedical Engineering* 48, no. 1 (2019): 92–103, https://doi.org/10.1007/s10439-019-02382-2.
8. T. J. Walilko, D. C. Viano, and C. A. Bir, "Biomechanics of the Head for Olympic Boxer Punches to the Face," *British Journal of Sports Medicine* 39 (2005): 710–19, https://doi.org/10.1136/bjsm.2004.014126.
9. Steven P. Broglio et al., "Cumulative Head Impact Burden in High School Football," *Journal of Neurotrauma* 28 (2011): 2069–78, https://doi.org/10.1089/neu.2011.1825; Steven P. Broglio et al., "Estimation of Head Impact Exposure in High School Football: Implications for Regulating Contact Practices," *American Journal of Sports Medicine* 41, no. 12 (2013): 2877–84, https://doi.org/10.1177/0363546513502458; Steven P. Broglio et al., "Football Players' Head-Impact Exposure after Limiting of Full-Contact Practices," *Journal of Athletic Training* 51, no. 7 (2016): 511–18, https://doi.org/10.4085/1062-6050-51.7.04; Joseph J. Crisco et al., "Head Impact Exposure in Collegiate Football Players," *Journal of Biomechanics* 44, no. 15 (2011): 2673–78, https://doi.org/10.1016/j.jbiomech.2011.08.003; Douglas Martini et al., "Subconcussive Head Impact Biomechanics: Comparing Differing Offensive Schemes," *Medicine & Science in Sports & Exercise* 45, no. 4 (2013): 755–61, https://doi.org/10.1249/MSS.0b013e3182798758; Jason P. Mihalik et al., "Measurement of Head Impacts in Collegiate Football Players: An Investigation of Positional and Event-Type Differences," *Neurosurgery* 61, no. 6 (2007): 1229–35, https://doi.org/10.1227/01.neu.0000306103.68635.1a.
10. Broglio et al., "Cumulative Head Impact Burden."
11. Crisco et al., "Head Impact Exposure."
12. Jonathan G. Beckwith et al., "Timing of Concussion Diagnosis Is Related to Head Impact Exposure Prior to Injury," *Medicine & Science in Sports & Exercise* 45, no. 4 (2014): 747–54, https://doi.org/10.1249/MSS.0b013e3182793067.
13. Ray W. Daniel, Steven Rowson, and Stefan M. Duma, "Head Impact Exposure in Youth Football: Middle School Ages 12–14 Years," *Journal of Biomechanical Engineering* 136, no. 9 (2014): 094501, https://doi.org/10.1115/1.4027872; Srinidhi Bellamkonda et al., "Head Impact Exposure in Practices Correlates with Exposure in Games for Youth Football Players," *Journal of Applied Biomechanics* 34, no. 5 (2018): 354–60, https://doi.org/10.1123/jab.2017-0207; Thayne A. Munce et al., "Head Impact Exposure and Neurologic Function of Youth Football Players," *Medicine & Science in Sports & Exercise* 47, no. 8 (2015): 1567–76, https://doi.org/10.1249/MSS.0000000000000591; Cobb et al., "Head Impact Exposure in Youth Football."

14. Bellamkonda et al., "Head Impact Exposure in Practices."

15. Ray W. Daniel, Steven Rowson, and Stefan M. Duma, "Head Impact Exposure in Youth Football," *Annals of Biomedical Engineering* 40, no. 4 (2012): 976–81, https://doi.org/10.1007/s10439-012-0530-7; Tyler J. Young et al., "Head Impact Exposure in Youth Football: Elementary School Ages 7-8 Years and the Effect of Returning Players," *Clinical Journal of Sport Medicine* 24, no. 4 (2014): 416–21, https://doi.org/10.1097/JSM.0000000000000055.

16. Ricky H. Wong, Andrew K. Wong, and Julian E. Bailes, "Frequency, Magnitude, and Distribution of Head Impacts in Pop Warner Football: The Cumulative Burden," *Clinical Neurology and Neurosurgery* 118 (2014): 1–4, https://doi.org/10.1016/j.clineuro.2013.11.036.

17. Tom Farrey, "Study Cites Youth Football for Issues," ESPN, January 28, 2015, https://www.espn.com/espn/otl/story/_/id/12243012/ex-nfl-players-played-tackle-football-youth-more-likely-thinking-memory-problems.

18. Ron Jadischke et al., "Quantitative and Qualitative Analysis of Head and Body Impacts in American 7v7 Non-tackle Football," *BMJ Open Sport & Exercise Medicine* 6, no. 1 (2020): e000638, https://doi.org/10.1136/bmjsem-2019-000638.

19. Robert C. Lynall et al., "A Comparison of Youth Flag and Tackle Football Head Impact Biomechanics," *Journal of Neurotrauma* 36 (2019): 1752–57, https://doi.org/10.1089/neu.2018.6236.

20. Lindley L. Brainard et al., "Gender Differences in Head Impacts Sustained by Collegiate Ice Hockey Players," *Medicine & Science in Sports & Exercise* 44, no. 2 (2012): 297–304, https://doi.org/10.1249/MSS.0b013e31822b0ab4; James T. Eckner et al., "Comparison of Head Impact Exposure between Male and Female High School Ice Hockey Athletes," *American Journal of Sports Medicine* 46, no. 9 (2018): 2253–62, https://doi.org/10.1177/0363546518777244; Bethany J. Wilcox et al., "Head Impact Exposure in Male and Female Collegiate Ice Hockey Players," *Journal of Biomechanics* 47 (2014): 109–14, https://doi.org/10.1016/j.jbiomech.2013.10.004.

21. Jason P. Mihalik et al., "Head Impact Biomechanics Differ between Girls and Boys Youth Ice Hockey Players," *Annals of Biomedical Engineering* 48, no. 1 (2019): 104–11, https://doi.org/10.1007/s10439-019-02343-9; N. Reed et al., "Measurement of Head Impacts in Youth Ice Hockey Players," *Orthopedics & Biomechanics* 31 (2010): 826–33, https://doi.org/10.1055/s-0030-1263103; Jason P. Mihalik et al., "Does Cervical Muscle Strength in Youth Ice Hockey Players Affect Head Impact Biomechanics?," *Clinical Journal of Sport Medicine* 21, no. 5 (2011): 416–21, https://doi.org/10.1097/JSM.0B013E31822C8A5C.

22. Lindsey C. Lamond et al., "Linear Acceleration in Direct Head Contact across Impact Type, Player Position, and Playing Scenario in Collegiate Women's Soccer Players," *Journal of Athletic Training* 53, no. 2 (2018): 115–21, https://doi.org/10.4085/1062-6050-90-17; Emily McCuen et al., "Collegiate Women's Soccer Players Suffer Greater Cumulative Head Impacts Than Their High School Counterparts," *Journal of Biomechanics* 48 (2015): 3720–23, https://doi.org/10.1016/j.jbiomech.2015.08.003; Jaclyn N. Press and Steven Rowson, "Quantifying Head Impact Exposure in Collegiate Women' s Soccer," *Clinical Journal of Sport Medicine* 27 (2017): 104–10, https://doi.org/10.1097/JSM.0000000000000313.

23. David H. Janda, Cynthia A. Bir, and Angela L. Cheney, "An Evaluation of the Cumulative Concussive Effect of Soccer Heading in the Youth Population," *Injury Control and Safety Promotion* 9, no. 1 (2002): 25–31, https://doi.org/10.1076/icsp.9.1.25.3324.

24. Doug King et al., "Head Impacts in a Junior Rugby League Team Measured with a Wireless Head Impact Sensor: An Exploratory Analysis," *Journal of Neurosurgery: Pediatrics* 19 (2017): 13–23, https://doi.org/10.3171/2016.7.PEDS1684; Doug A. King et al., "Similar Head Impact Acceleration Measured Using Instrumented Ear Patches in

a Junior Rugby Union Team during Matches in Comparison with Other Sports," *Journal of Neurosurgery: Pediatrics* 18 (2016): 65–72, https://doi.org/10.3171/2015.12.PEDS15 605.

25. Mark Hecimovich et al., "Youth Australian Footballers Experience Similar Impact Forces to the Head as Junior- and Senior-League Players: A Prospective Study of Kinematic Measurements," *Journal of Sports Science and Medicine* 17 (2018): 547–56.

26. Bryson B. Reynolds et al., "Comparative Analysis of Head Impact in Contact and Collision Sports," *Journal of Neurotrauma* 34 (2017): 38–49, https://doi.org/10.1089/neu.2015.4308.

27. Broglio et al., "Cumulative Head Impact Burden"; Broglio et al., "Estimation of Head Impact Exposure"; Broglio et al., "Football Players' Head-Impact Exposure"; Joseph J. Crisco et al., "Magnitude of Head Impact Exposures in Individual Collegiate Football Players," *Journal of Applied Biomechanics* 28, no. 2 (2013): 174–83, https://doi.org/10.1123/jab.28.2.174; Martini et al., "Subconcussive Head Impact Biomechanics"; Mihalik et al., "Measurement of Head Impacts"; Bryson B. Reynolds et al., "Practice Type Effects on Head Impact in Collegiate Football," *Journal of Neurosurgery* 124, no. February (2016): 501–10, https://doi.org/10.3171/2015.5.JNS15573; Jillian E. Urban et al., "Head Impact Exposure in Youth Football: High School Ages 14 to 18 Years and Cumulative Impact Analysis," *Annals of Biomedical Engineering* 41, no. 12 (2013): 2474–87, https://doi.org/10.1007/s10439-013-0861-z.

28. Sam Borden, Mika Gröndahl, and Joe Ward, "What Happened Within This Player's Skull," *New York Times*, January 9, 2017, https://www.nytimes.com/interactive/2017/01/09/sports/football/what-happened-within-this-players-skull-football-concussions.html?smid=tw-nytimes&smtyp=cur&_r=0.

29. Jonathan G. Beckwith et al., "Head Impact Exposure Sustained by Football Players on Days of Diagnosed Concussion," *Medicine & Science in Sports & Exercise* 45, no. 4 (2013): 737–46, https://doi.org/10.1249/MSS.0b013e3182792ed7.

30. Walilko, Viano, and Bir, "Biomechanics of the Head for Olympic Boxer Punches."

31. Cobb et al., "Head Impact Exposure in Youth Football"; Daniel, Rowson, and Duma, "Head Impact Exposure: Middle School"; Campolettano et al., "Development of a Concussion Risk Function"; Bellamkonda et al., "Head Impact Exposure in Practices"; Munce et al., "Head Impact Exposure and Neurologic Function"; Young et al., "Head Impact Exposure in Youth Football."

32. Mihalik et al., "Head Impact Biomechanics Differ."

33. Eckner et al., "Comparison of Head Impact Exposure"; Mihalik et al., "Does Cervical Muscle Strength"; Reed et al., "Measurement of Head Impacts"; Wilcox et al., "Head Impact Exposure"; Bethany J. Wilcox et al., "Biomechanics of Head Impacts Associated with Diagnosed Concussion in Female Collegiate Ice Hockey Players," *Journal of Biomechanics* 48 (2015): 2201–4, https://doi.org/10.1016/j.jbiomech.2015.04.005.

34. Erin M. Hanlon and Cynthia A. Bir, "Real-Time Head Acceleration Measurement in Girls' Youth Soccer," *Medicine & Science in Sports & Exercise* 44, no. 6 (2012): 1102–8, https://doi.org/10.1249/MSS.0b013e3182444d7d; Lamond et al., "Linear Acceleration"; McCuen et al., "Collegiate Women's Soccer Players"; Press and Rowson, "Quantifying Head Impact Exposure."

35. Sara P. D. Chrisman et al., "Head Impact Exposure in Youth Soccer and Variation by Age and Sex," *Clinical Journal of Sport Medicine* 29, no. 1 (2019): 3–10, https://doi.org/10.1097/JSM.0000000000000497.

36. King et al., "Head Impacts in a Junior Rugby League"; King et al., "Similar Head Impact Acceleration"; Hecimovich et al., "Youth Australian Footballers."

37. Broglio et al., "Cumulative Head Impact Burden"; Broglio et al., "Estimation of Head Impact Exposure"; Broglio et al., "Football Players' Head-Impact Exposure";

Campolettano et al., "Development of a Concussion Risk Function"; Mihalik et al., "Measurement of Head Impacts."

38. Lamond et al., "Linear Acceleration"; Press and Rowson, "Quantifying Head Impact Exposure."

39. Jason P. Mihalik et al., "Head Impact Biomechanics in Youth Hockey: Comparisons Across Playing Position, Event Types, and Impact Locations," *Annals of Biomedical Engineering* 40, no. 1 (2012): 141–49, https://doi.org/10.1007/s10439-011-0405-3.

40. Crisco et al., "Magnitude of Head Impact Exposures"; Martini et al., "Subconcussive Head Impact Biomechanics"; Urban et al., "Head Impact Exposure."

41. Campolettano et al., "Development of a Concussion Risk Function."

42. Daniel, Rowson, and Duma, "Head Impact Exposure in Youth Football."

43. Steven P. Broglio et al., "Biomechanical Properties of Concussions in High School Football," *Medicine & Science in Sports & Exercise* 42, no. 11 (2010): 2064–71, https://doi.org/10.1249/MSS.0b013e3181dd9156; Nicholas Burger et al., "Tackle Technique and Tackle-Related Injuries in High-Level South African Rugby Union Under-18 Players: Real-Match Video Analysis," *British Journal of Sports Medicine* 50 (2016): 932–38, https://doi.org/10.1136/bjsports-2015-095295.

44. Lamond et al., "Linear Acceleration."

45. Young et al., "Head Impact Exposure in Youth Football."

46. Campolettano et al., "Development of a Concussion Risk Function"; Ryan A. Gellner et al., "Are Specific Players More Likely to Be Involved in High-Magnitude Head Impacts in Youth Football?," *Journal of Neurosurgery: Pediatrics* 24, no. 1 (2019): 47–53, https://doi.org/10.3171/2019.2.PEDS18176.

47. Mireille E. Kelley et al., "Physical Performance Measures Correlate with Head Impact Exposure in Youth Football," *Medicine & Science in Sports & Exercise* 52, no. 2 (2020): 449–56, https://doi.org/10.1249/MSS.0000000000002144.

48. Jaclyn Alois et al., "Do American Youth Football Players Intentionally Use Their Heads for High-Magnitude Impacts?," *American Journal of Sports Medicine* 47, no. 14 (2011): 3498–3504, https://doi.org/10.1177/0363546519882034.

49. Julianne D. Schmidt et al., "Safe-Play Knowledge, Aggression, and Head-Impact Biomechanics in Adolescent Ice Hockey Players," *Journal of Athletic Training* 51, no. 5 (2016): 366–72, https://doi.org/10.4085/1062-6050-51.5.04.

50. Martini et al., "Subconcussive Head Impact Biomechanics."

51. Mireille E. Kelley et al., "Comparison of Head Impact Exposure in Practice Drills among Multiple Youth Football Teams," *Journal of Neurosurgery: Pediatrics* 23 (2019): 381–89, https://doi.org/10.3171/2018.9.PEDS18314; Eamon T. Campolettano, Steven Rowson, and Stefan M. Duma, "Drill-Specific Head Impact Exposure in Youth Football Practice," *Journal of Neurosurgery: Pediatrics* 18 (2016): 536–41, https://doi.org/10.3171/2016.5.PEDS1696.

5. WHY THE YOUNG BRAIN IS VULNERABLE

1. Farrey, "Study Cites Youth Football for Issues."

2. Sandra Ackerman, *Discovering the Brain* (Washington DC: National Academies Press, 1992), https://www.ncbi.nlm.nih.gov/books/NBK234146/.

3. Jay N. Giedd et al., "Brain Development during Childhood and Adolescence: A Longitudinal MRI Study," *Nature Neuroscience* 2, no. 10 (1999): 861–63, https://doi.org/10.1038/13158.

4. Ackerman, *Discovering the Brain*.

5. Thomas M. Reeves, Linda L. Phillips, and John T. Povlishock, "Myelinated and Unmyelinated Axons of the Corpus Callosum Differ in Vulnerability and Functional Recovery following Traumatic Brain Injury," *Experimental Neurology* 196, no. 1 (2005): 126–37, https://doi.org/10.1016/j.expneurol.2005.07.014; Thomas M. Reeves et al., "Unmyelinated Axons Show Selective Rostrocaudal Pathology in the Corpus Callosum after Traumatic Brain Injury," *Journal of Neuropathology and Experimental Neurology* 71, no. 3 (2012): 198–210, https://doi.org/10.1097/NEN.0b013e3182482590.

6. Ackerman, *Discovering the Brain*.

7. Philip Shaw et al., "Neurodevelopmental Trajectories of the Human Cerebral Cortex," *Journal of Neuroscience* 28, no. 14 (2008): 3586–94, https://doi.org/10.1523/JNEUROSCI.5309-07.2008.

8. Sarah-Jayne Blakemore and Suparna Choudhury, "Development of the Adolescent Brain: Implications for Executive Function and Social Cognition," *Journal of Child Psychology and Psychiatry* 47, no. 3–4 (2006): 296–312, https://doi.org/10.1111/j.1469-7610.2006.01611.x.

9. Nitin Gogtay and Paul M. Thompson, "Mapping Gray Matter Development: Implications for Typical Development and Vulnerability to Psychopathology," *Brain and Cognition* 72, no. 1 (2010): 6–15, https://doi.org/10.1016/j.bandc.2009.08.009.

10. Ackerman, *Discovering the Brain*.

11. Giedd et al., "Brain Development during Childhood and Adolescence."

12. Jon Bardin, "Unlocking the Brain," *Nature* 487, no. 7405 (2012): 24–26, https://doi.org/10.1038/487024a; Fulton Crews, Jun He, and Clyde Hodge, "Adolescent Cortical Development: A Critical Period of Vulnerability for Addiction," *Pharmacology, Biochemistry and Behavior* 86, no. 2 (2007): 189–99, https://doi.org/10.1016/j.pbb.2006.12.001.

13. Beatriz Luna et al., "Maturation of Cognitive Processes from Late Childhood to Adulthood," *Child Development* 75, no. 5 (2004): 1357–72, https://doi.org/10.1111/j.1467-8624.2004.00745.x.

14. Blakemore and Choudhury, "Development of the Adolescent Brain"; Luna et al., "Maturation of Cognitive Processes."

15. Michael D. De Bellis et al., "Developmental Traumatology Part II: Brain Development," *Biological Psychiatry* 45, no. 10 (1999): 1271–84.

16. Crews, He, and Hodge, "Adolescent Cortical Development."

17. Blakemore and Choudhury, "Development of the Adolescent Brain."

18. Giedd et al., "Brain Development during Childhood and Adolescence"; Rhoshel K. Lenroot and Jay N. Giedd, "Brain Development in Children and Adolescents: Insights from Anatomical Magnetic Resonance Imaging," *Neuroscience and Biobehavioral Reviews* 30, no. 6 (2006): 718–29, https://doi.org/10.1016/j.neubiorev.2006.06.001; Robert W. Thatcher, "Maturation of the Human Frontal Lobes: Physiological Evidence for Staging," *Developmental Neuropsychology* 7, no. 3 (1991): 397–419, https://doi.org/10.1080/87565649109540500.

19. Ackerman, *Discovering the Brain*.

20. Lindsay Snook et al., "Diffusion Tensor Imaging of Neurodevelopment in Children and Young Adults," *NeuroImage* 26, no. 4 (2005): 1164–73, https://doi.org/10.1016/j.neuroimage.2005.03.016.

21. Fidel Hernandez et al., "Lateral Impacts Correlate with Falx Cerebri Displacement and Corpus Callosum Trauma in Sports-Related Concussions," *Biomechanics and Modeling in Mechanobiology* 18, no. 3 (2019): 631–49, https://doi.org/10.1007/s10237-018-01106-0.

22. Ackerman, *Discovering the Brain*.

23. Akiko Uematsu et al., "Developmental Trajectories of Amygdala and Hippocampus from Infancy to Early Adulthood in Healthy Individuals," *PLOS ONE* 7, no. 10 (2012): e46970, https://doi.org/10.1371/journal.pone.0046970.

24. Uematsu et al., "Developmental Trajectories"

25. Gogtay and Thompson, "Mapping Gray Matter Development"; Lenroot and Giedd, "Brain Development in Children and Adolescents."

26. Blakemore and Choudhury, "Development of the Adolescent Brain."

27. Herman T. Epstein, "Stages of Increased Cerebral Blood Flow Accompany Stages of Rapid Brain Growth," *Brain & Development* 21, no. 8 (1999): 535–39.

28. Gerald E. Schneider, "Is It Really Better to Have Your Brain Lesion Early? A Revision of the 'Kennard Principle,'" *Neuropsychologia* 17, no. 6 (1979): 557–83, https://doi.org/10.1016/0028-3932(79)90033-2.

29. Francesca Cacucci and Faraneh Vargha-Khadem, "Contributions of Nonhuman Primate Research to Understanding the Consequences of Human Brain Injury during Development," *PNAS* 116, no. 52 (2019): 26204–9, https://doi.org/10.1073/pnas.1912952116.

30. Bryan Kolb and Ian Q. Whishaw, "Brain Plasticity and Behavior," *Annual Review of Psychology* 49, no. 1 (1998): 43–64, https://doi.org/10.1146/annurev.psych.49.1.43.

31. Mark H. Johnson and Michelle De Haan, *Developmental Cognitive Neuroscience: An Introduction* (Chichester, UK: Wiley Blackwell, 2015); Shalini Narayana et al., "Neuroimaging and Neuropsychological Studies in Sports-Related Concussions in Adolescents: Current State and Future Directions," *Frontiers in Neurology* 10 (2019): 1–10, https://doi.org/10.3389/fneur.2019.00538.

32. Daniel W. Shrey, Grace S. Griesbach, and Christopher C. Giza, "The Pathophysiology of Concussions in Youth," *Physical Medicine & Rehabilitation Clinics of North America* 22, no. 4 (2012): 577–602, https://doi.org/10.1016/j.pmr.2011.08.002; Elisabeth A. Wilde, Jill V. Hunter, and Erin D. Bigler, "Pediatric Traumatic Brain Injury: Neuroimaging and Neurorehabilitation Outcome," *NeuroRehabilitation* 31, no. 3 (2012): 245–60, https://doi.org/10.3233/NRE-2012-0794.

33. Cacucci and Vargha-Khadem, "Contributions of Nonhuman Primate Research"; Kevin M. Guskiewicz and Tamara C. Valovich Mcleod, "Pediatric Sports-Related Concussion," *PM&R* 3, no. 4 (2011): 353–64, https://doi.org/10.1016/j.pmrj.2010.12.006; Shrey, Griesbach, and Giza, "Pathophysiology of Concussions."

34. Crews, He, and Hodge, "Adolescent Cortical Development."

35. Jürgen Hänggi et al., "Structural Neuroplasticity in the Sensorimotor Network of Professional Female Ballet Dancers," *Human Brain Mapping* 31, no. 8 (2010): 1196–1206, https://doi.org/10.1002/hbm.20928.

36. Cacucci and Vargha-Khadem, "Contributions of Nonhuman Primate Research"; Vicki Anderson, Megan Spencer-Smith, and Amanda Wood, "Do Children Really Recover Better? Neurobehavioural Plasticity after Early Brain Insult," *Brain* 134, no. 8 (2011): 2197–2221, https://doi.org/10.1093/brain/awr103; Susan L. Andersen and Martin H. Teicher, "Stress, Sensitive Periods and Maturational Events in Adolescent Depression," *Trends in Neurosciences* 31, no. 4 (2008): 183–91, https://doi.org/10.1016/j.tins.2008.01.004.

37. Bardin, "Unlocking the Brain."

38. M. M. Stephens, L. C. S. Hsu, and J. C. Y. Leong, "Leg Length Discrepancy after Femoral Shaft Fractures in Children: Review after Skeletal Maturity," *Journal of Bone and Joint Surgery (British)* 71, no. 4 (1989): 615–18.

39. Marie-Lyne Nault and James Kasser, "Evaluation and Management of Pediatric Femur Fractures," in *Pediatric Femur Fractures*, ed. Daniel J. Hedequist and Benton E. Heyworth, 215–28 (Boston, MA: Springer, 2016).

40. M. J. Herring et al., "Growth of Alveoli during Postnatal Development in Humans Based on Stereological Estimation," *American Journal of Physiology Lung Cellular and Molecular Physiology* 307, no. 4 (2014): L338–44, https://doi.org/10.1152/ajplung.00094.2014.

41. Diane R. Gold et al., "Effects of Cigarette Smoking on Lung Function in Adolescent Boys and Girls," *New England Journal of Medicine* 335, no. 13 (1996): 931–37.

42. John K. Wiencke and Karl T. Kelsey, "Teen Smoking, Field Cancerization, and a 'Critical Period' Hypothesis for Lung Cancer Susceptibility," *Environmental Health Perspectives* 110, no. 6 (2002): 555–58.

43. Ayer et al., "Lifetime Risk."

44. Johanna M. Meulepas et al., "Radiation Exposure from Pediatric CT Scans and Subsequent Cancer Risk in the Netherlands," *JNCI: Journal of the National Cancer Institute* 111, no. 3 (2019): 256–64, https://doi.org/10.1093/jnci/djy104.

45. Cynthia A. Riccio and Jeremy R. Sullivan, *Pediatric Neurotoxicology* (Cham, Switzerland: Springer International, 2016).

46. Crews, He, and Hodge, "Adolescent Cortical Development."

47. Grace Blest-Hopley et al., "Disrupted Parahippocampal and Midbrain Function Underlie Slower Verbal Learning in Adolescent-Onset Regular Cannabis Use," *Psychopharmacology* (2019), https://doi.org/10.1007/s00213-019-05407-9; Joanna Jacobus et al., "Cortical Thickness in Adolescent Marijuana and Alcohol Users: A Three-Year Prospective Study from Adolescence to Young Adulthood," *Developmental Cognitive Neuroscience* 16 (2015): 101–9, https://doi.org/10.1016/j.dcn.2015.04.006.

48. Andersen and Teicher, "Stress, Sensitive Periods and Maturational Events"; Gene H. Brody et al., "Protective Prevention Effects on the Association of Poverty with Brain Development," *JAMA Pediatrics* 171, no. 1 (2017): 46–52, https://doi.org/10.1001/jamapediatrics.2016.2988; Cacucci and Vargha-Khadem, "Contributions of Nonhuman Primate Research."

49. Katie A. McLaughlin, David Weissman, and Debbie Bitrán, "Childhood Adversity and Neural Development: A Systematic Review," *Annual Review of Developmental Psychology* 1 (2019): 277–312, https://doi.org/10.1146/annurev-devpsych-121318-084950.

50. Andersen and Teicher, "Stress, Sensitive Periods and Maturational Events."

51. Luciana, "Adolescent Brain"; Crews, He, and Hodge, "Adolescent Cortical Development."

52. Anderson, Spencer-Smith, and Wood, "Do Children Really Recover Better?"

6. WHY IT'S NOT ALL ABOUT CONCUSSIONS

1. Rich Barlow, "BU-Led Study: CTE May Occur without Concussions," *Brink: Pioneering Research from Boston University*, January 18, 2018, http://www.bu.edu/articles/2018/cte-caused-by-head-injuries/.

2. Centers for Disease Control and Prevention, "What Is a Concussion?," Heads Up, February 12, 2019, https://www.cdc.gov/headsup/basics/concussion_whatis.html.

3. Narayana et al., "Neuroimaging and Neuropsychological Studies."

4. Clifford A. Robbins et al., "Self-Reported Concussion History: Impact of Providing a Definition of Concussion," *Open Access Journal of Sports Medicine* 5 (2014): 99–103, https://doi.org/10.2147/OAJSM.S58005.

5. Dionissios T. Hristopulos et al., "Disrupted Information Flow in Resting-State in Adolescents with Sports Related Concussion," *Frontiers in Human Neuroscience* 13 (2019): 419, https://doi.org/10.3389/fnhum.2019.00419; Narayana et al., "Neuroimaging and Neuropsychological Studies"; Sourajit M. Mustafi et al., "Acute White-Matter Abnormalities in Sports-Related Concussion: A Diffusion Tensor Imaging Study," *Journal of Neurotrauma* 35, no. 22 (2018): 2653–64, https://doi.org/10.1089/neu.2017.5158.

6. Zachary Y. Kerr et al., "Concussion Rates in U.S. Middle School Athletes, 2015–2016 School Year," *American Journal of Preventive Medicine* 53, no. 6 (2017): 914–18, https://doi.org/10.1016/j.amepre.2017.05.017; Zachary Y. Kerr et al., "Concussion Incidence and Trends in 20 High School Sports," *Pediatrics* 144, no. 5 (2019): e20192180, https://doi.org/10.1542/peds.2019-2180; Joseph A. Rosenthal et al., "National High School Athlete Concussion Rates from 2005–2006 to 2011–2012," *American Journal of Sports Medicine* 42, no. 7 (2014): 1710–15, https://doi.org/10.1177/0363546514530091.

7. Sara P. D. Chrisman et al., "Concussion Incidence, Duration, and Return to School and Sport in 5- to 14-Year-Old American Football Athletes," *Journal of Pediatrics* 207 (2018): 176–84, https://doi.org/10.1016/j.jpeds.2018.11.003.

8. Thomas P. Dompier et al., "Incidence of Concussion during Practice and Games in Youth, High School, and Collegiate American Football Players," *JAMA Pediatrics* 169, no. 7 (2015): 659–65, https://doi.org/10.1001/jamapediatrics.2015.0210.

9. Amanda M. Black et al., "The Risk of Injury Associated with Body Checking among Pee Wee Ice Hockey Players: An Evaluation of Hockey Canada's National Body Checking Policy Change," *British Journal of Sports Medicine* 51 (2017): 1767–72, https://doi.org/10.1136/bjsports-2016-097392.

10. Kerr et al., "Concussion Rates in U.S. Middle School Athletes"; John W. O'Kane et al., "Concussion among Female Middle-School Soccer Players," *JAMA Pediatrics* 168, no. 3 (2019): 258–64, https://doi.org/10.1001/jamapediatrics.2013.4518; Kerr et al., "Concussion Incidence and Trends in 20 High School Sports."

11. Zachary Y. Kerr et al., "Injury Incidence in Youth, High School, and NCAA Men's Lacrosse," *Pediatrics* 143, no. 6 (2019): e20183482, https://doi.org/10.1542/peds.2018-3482; Zachary Y. Kerr et al., "Epidemiology of Youth Boys' and Girls' Lacrosse Injuries in the 2015 to 2016 Seasons," *Medicine & Science in Sports & Exercise* 50, no. 2 (2017): 284–91, https://doi.org/10.1249/MSS.0000000000001422.

12. Felix T. Leung et al., "Epidemiology of Injuries in Australian School Level Rugby Union," *Journal of Science and Medicine in Sport* 20, no. 8 (2017): 740–44, https://doi.org/10.1016/j.jsams.2017.03.006.

13. Mark D. Hecimovich and Doug King, "Prevalence of Head Injury and Medically Diagnosed Concussion in Junior-Level Community-Based Australian Rules Football," *Journal of Pediatrics and Child Health* 53 (2017): 246–51, https://doi.org/10.1111/jpc.13405.

14. Abigail C. Bretzin et al., "Sex Differences in the Clinical Incidence of Concussions, Missed School Days, and Time Loss in High School Student-Athletes," *American Journal of Sports Medicine* 46, no. 9 (2018): 2263–69, https://doi.org/10.1177/0363546518778251; Kerr et al., "Concussion Rates in U.S. Middle School Athletes."

15. Mihalik et al., "Head Impact Biomechanics Differ."

16. Bretzin et al., "Sex Differences in the Clinical Incidence of Concussions."

17. Kroshus et al., "Concussion Reporting, Sex, and Conformity."

18. Scott L. Zuckerman et al., "Epidemiology of Sports-Related Concussion in NCAA Athletes from 2009–2010 to 2013–2014," *American Journal of Sports Medicine* 43, no. 11 (2015): 2654–62, https://doi.org/10.1177/0363546515599634; Robert C. Lynall et al., "Concussion Mechanisms and Activities in Youth, High School, and College

Football," *Journal of Neurotrauma* 24 (2017): 2684–90, https://doi.org/10.1089/neu.2017.5032.

19. Andrew Watson, Jeffrey M. Mjaanes, and Council on Sports Medicine and Fitness, "Soccer Injuries in Children and Adolescents," *Pediatrics* 144, no. 5 (2019): e20192759, https://doi.org/10.1542/peds.2019-2759.

20. Kerr et al., "Concussion Incidence and Trends in 20 High School Sports"; Kerr et al., "Concussion Rates in U.S. Middle School Athletes"; Zuckerman et al., "Epidemiology of Sports-Related Concussion."

21. Steven Rowson et al., "Correlation of Concussion Symptom Profile with Head Impact Biomechanics: A Case for Individual-Specific Injury Tolerance," *Journal of Neurotrauma* 35, no. 4 (2018): 681–90, https://doi.org/10.1089/neu.2017.5169.

22. Beckwith et al., "Timing of Concussion Diagnosis"; Broglio et al., "Biomechanical Properties."

23. Campolettano et al., "Development of a Concussion Risk Function."

24. Centers for Disease Control and Prevention, "What Is a Concussion?"

25. Johna K. Register-Mihalik et al., "Considerations for Athletic Trainers: A Review of Guidance on Mild Traumatic Brain Injury among Children from the Centers for Disease Control and Prevention and the National Athletic Trainers' Association," *Journal of Athletic Training* 54, no. 1 (2019): 12–20, https://doi.org/10.4085/1062-6050-451-18.

26. Jenna T. Reece et al., "A Biomarker for Concussion: The Good, the Bad, and the Unknown," *JALM* 5, no. 1 (2018): 170–82, https://doi.org/10.1093/jalm.2019.031187.

27. Breton M. Asken et al., "Immediate Removal from Activity after Sport-Related Concussion Is Associated with Shorter Clinical Recovery and Less Severe Symptoms in Collegiate Student-Athletes," *American Journal of Sports Medicine* 46, no. 6 (2018): 1465–74, https://doi.org/10.1177/0363546518757984; Daniel B. Charek et al., "Preliminary Evidence of a Dose-Response for Continuing to Play on Recovery Time after Concussion," *Journal of Head Trauma Rehabilitation* 35, no. 2 (2020): 85–91, https://doi.org/10.1097/HTR.0000000000000476.

28. Register-Mihalik et al., "Considerations for Athletic Trainers."

29. Stephen Kara et al., "Less Than Half of Patients Recover within 2 Weeks of Injury after a Sports-Related Mild Traumatic Brain Injury: A 2-Year Prospective Study," *Clinical Journal of Sport Medicine* 30, no. 2 (2020): 96–101, https://doi.org/10.1097/JSM.0000000000000811.

30. Michael McCrea et al., "Return to Play and Risk of Repeat Concussion in Collegiate Football Players: Comparative Analysis from the NCAA Concussion Study (1999–2001) and CARE Consortium (2014–2017)," *British Journal of Sports Medicine* 54, no. 2 (2019): 102–9, https://doi.org/10.1136/bjsports-2019-100579.

31. Matthew A. Eisenberg et al., "Time Interval between Concussions and Symptom Duration," *Pediatrics* 132 (2013): 8–17, https://doi.org/10.1542/peds.2013-0432.

32. Landon B. Lempke et al., "Examination of Reaction Time Deficits following Concussion: A Systematic Review and Meta-Analysis," *Sports Medicine* 50, no. 7 (2020): 1341–59, https://doi.org/10.1007/s40279-020-01281-0; Amanda L. McGowan et al., "Acute and Protracted Disruptions to Inhibitory Control following Sports-Related Concussion," *Neuropsychologia* 131 (2019): 223–32, https://doi.org/10.1016/j.neuropsychologia.2019.05.026.

33. Anthony P. Kontos et al., "Recovery following Sport-Related Concussion: Integrating Pre- and Postinjury Factors into Multidisciplinary Care," *Journal of Head Trauma Rehabilitation* 34, no. 6 (2019): 394–401, https://doi.org/10.1097/HTR.0000000000000536.

34. Eisenberg et al., "Time Interval."

35. Kate Berz et al., "Sex-Specific Differences in the Severity of Symptoms and Recovery Rate following Sports-Related Concussion in Young Athletes," *Physician and*

Sportsmedicine 41, no. 2 (2013): 58–63, https://doi.org/10.3810/psm.2013.05.2015; Bretzin et al., "Sex Differences in the Clinical Incidence of Concussions"; Kara et al., "Less Than Half of Patients Recover."

36. Narayana et al., "Neuroimaging and Neuropsychological Studies."

37. Nathan W. Churchill et al., "Mapping Brain Recovery after Concussion: From Acute Injury to 1 Year after Medical Clearance," *Neurology* 93, no. 21 (2019): e1980–92, https://doi.org/10.1212/WNL.0000000000008523; Michelle L. Keightley et al., "Is There Evidence for Neurodegenerative Change following Traumatic Brain Injury in Children and Youth? A Scoping Review," *Frontiers in Human Neuroscience* 8, no. 139 (2014), https://doi.org/10.3389/fnhum.2014.00139.

38. Lempke et al., "Examination of Reaction Time Deficits"; McGowan et al., "Acute and Protracted Disruptions."

39. M. Alison Brooks et al., "Concussion Increases Odds of Sustaining a Lower Extremity Musculoskeletal Injury after Return to Play among Collegiate Athletes," *American Journal of Sports Medicine* 44, no. 3 (2016): 742–47, https://doi.org/10.1177/0363546515622387; April L. McPherson et al., "Effect of a Concussion on Anterior Cruciate Ligament Injury Risk in a General Population," *Sports Medicine* 50, no. 6 (2020): 1203–10, https://doi.org/10.1007/s40279-020-01262-3.

40. Aaron M. Karlin, "Concussion in the Pediatric and Adolescent Population: 'Different Population, Different Concerns,'" *PM&R* 3, no. 10 Suppl 2 (2011): S369–79, https://doi.org/10.1016/j.pmrj.2011.07.015; Zachary Y. Kerr et al., "Concussion Symptoms and Return to Play Time in Youth, High School, and College American Football Athletes," *JAMA Pediatrics* 170, no. 7 (2016): 647–53, https://doi.org/10.1001/jamapediatrics.2016.0073.

41. Karlin, "Concussion in the Pediatric and Adolescent Population."

42. Nicole L. Hoffman et al., "Influence of Postconcussion Sleep Duration on Concussion Recovery in Collegiate Athletes," *Clinical Journal of Sport Medicine* 30, Suppl 1 (2020): S29–35, https://doi.org/10.1097/JSM.0000000000000538.

43. Carol DeMatteo et al., "Effectiveness of Return to Activity and Return to School Protocols for Children Postconcussion: A Systematic Review," *BMJ Open Sport & Exercise Medicine* 6 (2020): e000667, https://doi.org/10.1136/bmjsem-2019-000667.

44. Register-Mihalik et al., "Considerations for Athletic Trainers."

45. William T. Tsushima et al., "Invalid Baseline Testing with ImPACT: Does Sandbagging Occur with High School Athletes?," *Applied Neuropsychology: Child* (2019): 1–10, https://doi.org/10.1080/21622965.2019.1642202.

46. Annie Baillargeon et al., "Neuropsychological and Neurophysiological Assessment of Sport Concussion in Children, Adolescents and Adults," *Brain Injury* 26, no. 3 (2012): 211–20, https://doi.org/10.3109/02699052.2012.654590; Guskiewicz and Valovich Mcleod, "Pediatric Sports-Related Concussion"; Scott L. Zuckerman et al., "Recovery from Sports-Related Concussion: Days to Return to Neurocognitive Baseline in Adolescents versus Young Adults," *Surgical Neurology International* 3 (2012): 130, https://doi.org/10.4103/2152-7806.102945.

47. Narayana et al., "Neuroimaging and Neuropsychological Studies"; Douglas P. Terry et al., "FMRI Hypoactivation during Verbal Learning and Memory in Former High School Football Players with Multiple Concussions," *Archives of Clinical Neuropsychology* 30 (2015): 341–55, https://doi.org/10.1093/arclin/acv020.

48. Ikbeom Jang et al., "Every Hit Matters: White Matter Diffusivity Changes in High School Football Athletes Are Correlated with Repetitive Head Acceleration Event Exposure," *NeuroImage: Clinical* 24 (2019): 101930, https://doi.org/10.1016/j.nicl.2019.101930; Inga K. Koerte et al., "A Prospective Study of Physician-Observed Concussion during a Varsity University Hockey Season: White Matter Integrity in Ice Hockey Players. Part 3 of 4," *Neurosurgical Focus* 33, no. 6 (2012): 1–7, https://doi.org/10.3171/2012.10.focus12303.

49. Jeffrey J. Bazarian et al., "Persistent, Long-Term Cerebral White Matter Changes after Sports-Related Repetitive Head Impacts," *PLOS ONE* 9, no. 4 (2014): e94734, https://doi.org/10.1371/journal.pone.0094734.

50. Naeim Bahrami et al., "Subconcussive Head Impact Exposure and White Matter Tract Changes over a Single Season of Youth Football," *Radiology* 281, no. 3 (2016): 919–26, https://doi.org/10.1148/radiol.2016160564.

51. Kausar Abbas et al., "Effects of Repetitive Sub-concussive Brain Injury on the Functional Connectivity of Default Mode Network in High School Football Athletes," *Developmental Neuropsychology* 40, no. 1 (2015): 51–56, https://doi.org/10.1080/87565641.2014.990455; Gowtham Murugesan et al., "Changes in Resting State MRI Networks from a Single Season of Football Distinguishes Controls, Low, and High Head Impact Exposure," *Proceedings: IEEE International Symposium on Biomedical Imaging* (2017): 464–67, https://doi.org/10.1109/ISBI.2017.7950561; Semyon M. Slobounov et al., "The Effect of Repetitive Subconcussive Collisions on Brain Integrity in Collegiate Football Players over a Single Football Season: A Multi-modal Neuroimaging Study," *NeuroImage: Clinical* 14 (2017): 708–18, https://doi.org/10.1016/j.nicl.2017.03.006.

52. "Playing Youth Football Could Affect Brain Development," Radiological Society of North America, November 26, 2018, https://press.rsna.org/timssnet/media/pressreleases/14_pr_target.cfm?ID=2051.

53. Diana O. Svaldi et al., "Cerebrovascular Reactivity Changes in Asymptomatic Female Athletes Attributable to High School Soccer Participation," *Brain Imaging and Behavior* 11 (2017): 98–112, https://doi.org/10.1007/s11682-016-9509-6.

54. Allen A. Champagne et al., "Changes in Volumetric and Metabolic Parameters Relate to Differences in Exposure to Sub-concussive Head Impacts," *Journal of Cerebral Blood Flow & Metabolism* 40, no. 7 (2020): 1453–67, https://doi.org/10.1177/0271678X19862861.

55. Sumra Bari et al., "Dependence on Subconcussive Impacts of Brain Metabolism in Collision Sport Athletes: An MR Spectroscopic Study," *Brain Imaging and Behavior* 13, no. 3 (2019): 735–49, https://doi.org/10.1007/s11682-018-9861-9; Bazarian et al., "Persistent, Long-Term Cerebral White Matter Changes"; Jonathan M. Oliver et al., "Fluctuations in Blood Biomarkers of Head Trauma in NCAA Football Athletes over the Course of a Season," *Journal of Neurosurgery* 30, no. 5 (2019): 1656–62, https://doi.org/10.3171/2017.12.JNS172035.

56. Itai Weissberg et al., "Imaging Blood-Brain Barrier Dysfunction in Football Players," *JAMA Neurology* 71, no. 11 (2014): 1453–55.

57. Brian Johnson et al., "Effects of Subconcussive Head Trauma on the Default Mode Network of the Brain," *Journal of Neurotrauma* 31, no. 23 (2014): 1907–13, https://doi.org/10.1089/neu.2014.3415.

58. Jaclyn B. Caccese et al., "Postural Control Deficits after Repetitive Soccer Heading," *Clinical Journal of Sport Medicine* (2018): 1–7, https://doi.org/10.1097/JSM.0000000000000709; Thomas Di Virgilio et al., "Evidence for Acute Electrophysiological and Cognitive Changes following Routine Soccer Heading," *EBioMedicine* 13 (2016): 66–71, https://doi.org/10.1016/j.ebiom.2016.10.029.

59. James T. Eckner et al., "Effect of Routine Sport Participation on Short-Term Clinical Neurological Outcomes: A Comparison of Non-contact, Contact, and Collision Sport Athletes," *Sports Medicine* 50 (2019): 1027–38, https://doi.org/10.1007/s40279-019-01200-y; Benjamin L. Brett and Gary S. Solomon, "Comparison of Neurocognitive Performance in Contact and Noncontact Nonconcussed High School Athletes across a Two-Year Interval," *Developmental Neuropsychology* 42, no. 2 (2017): 70–82, https://doi.org/10.1080/87565641.2016.1243114.

60. Jaclyn B. Caccese et al., "Effects of Repetitive Head Impacts on a Concussion Assessment Battery," *Medicine & Science in Sports & Exercise* 51, no. 7 (2019):

1355–61, https://doi.org/10.1249/MSS.000000000001905; Munce et al., "Head Impact Exposure and Neurologic Function."

61. Inga K. Koerte et al., "Impaired Cognitive Performance in Youth Athletes Exposed to Repetitive Head Impacts," *Journal of Neurotrauma* 34 (2017): 2389–95, https://doi.org/10.1089/neu.2016.4960; Eckner et al., "Effect of Routine Sport Participation."

62. Bari et al., "Dependence on Subconcussive Impacts"; Champagne et al., "Changes in Volumetric and Metabolic Parameters"; Michael L. Lipton et al., "Soccer Heading Associated with White Matter Microstructural and Cognitive Abnormalities," *Radiology* 268, no. 3 (2013): 850–57, https://doi.org/10.1148/radiol.13130545.

63. Koerte et al., "Impaired Cognitive Performance"; Walter F. Stewart et al., "Heading Frequency Is More Strongly Related to Cognitive Performance Than Unintentional Head Impacts in Amateur Soccer Players," *Frontiers in Neurology* 9, no. 240 (2018): 1–10, https://doi.org/10.3389/fneur.2018.00240.

64. Daniel R. Seichepine et al., "Profile of Self-Reported Problems with Executive Functioning in College and Professional Football Players," *Journal of Neurotrauma* 30, no. 14 (2013): 1299–1304, https://doi.org/10.1089/neu.2012.2690; Christian Lepage et al., "Limbic System Structure Volumes and Associated Neurocognitive Functioning in Former NFL Players," *Brain Imaging and Behavior* 13, no. 3 (2018): 725–34, https://doi.org/10.1007/s11682-018-9895-z.

65. Xavier Guell et al., "Functional Connectivity Changes in Retired Rugby League Players: A Data-Driven Functional Magnetic Resonance Imaging Study," *Journal of Neurotrauma* 37, no. 16 (2020): 1788–96, https://doi.org/10.1089/neu.2019.6782; Adam Hampshire, Alex MacDonald, and Adrian M. Owen, "Hypoconnectivity and Hyperfrontality in Retired American Football Players," *Scientific Reports* 3 (2013): 2972, https://doi.org/10.1038/srep02972; John Hart Jr. et al., "Neuroimaging of Cognitive Dysfunction and Depression in Aging Retired National Football League Players," *JAMA Neurology* 70, no. 3 (2013): 326–35, https://doi.org/10.1001/2013.jamaneurol. 340; Inga K. Koerte et al., "White Matter Integrity in the Brains of Professional Soccer Players without a Symptomatic Concussion," *JAMA* 308, no. 18 (2012): 1859–61, https://doi.org/10.1001/jama.2012.13735; Inga K. Koerte et al., "Cortical Thinning in Former Professional Soccer Players," *Brain Imaging and Behavior* 10 (2016): 792–98, https://doi.org/10.1007/s11682-015-9442-0.

66. Philip H. Montenigro et al., "Cumulative Head Impact Exposure Predicts Later-Life Depression, Apathy, Executive Dysfunction, and Cognitive Impairment in Former High School and College Football Players," *Journal of Neurotrauma* 34 (2017): 328–40, https://doi.org/10.1089/neu.2016.4413.

67. William T. Tsushima et al., "Are There Subconcussive Neuropsychological Effects in Youth Sports? An Exploratory Study of High- and Low-Contact Sports," *Applied Neuropsychology: Child* 5, no. 2 (2016): 149–55, https://doi.org/10.1080/21622965.2015.1052813; William T. Tsushima et al., "Effects of Repetitive Subconcussive Head Trauma on the Neuropsychological Test Performance of High School Athletes: A Comparison of High, Moderate, and Low Contact Sports," *Applied Neuropsychology: Child* 8, no. 3 (2019): 223–30, https://doi.org/10.1080/21622965.2018. 1427095.

68. William T. Tsushima et al., "Computerized Neuropsychological Test Performance of Youth Football Players at Different Positions: A Comparison of High and Low Contact Players," *Applied Neuropsychology: Child* 7, no. 3 (2018): 217–23, https://doi.org/10.1080/21622965.2017.1290530.

69. Adam D. Bohr, Jason D. Boardman, and Matthew B. McQueen, "Association of Adolescent Sport Participation with Cognition and Depressive Symptoms in Early Adulthood," *Orthopaedic Journal of Sports Medicine* 7, no. 9 (2019): 1–11, https://doi.org/10.1177/2325967119868658; Sameer K. Deshpande et al., "The Association be-

tween Adolescent Football Participation and Early Adulthood Depression," *PLOS ONE* 15, no. 3 (2020): e0229978, https://doi.org/10.1371/journal.pone.0229978.

70. Deshpande et al., "Association between Adolescent Football Participation."
71. Beckwith et al., "Head Impact Exposure Sustained by Football Players"; Steven P. Broglio et al., "Head Impact Density: A Model to Explain the Elusive Concussion Threshold," *Journal of Neurotrauma* 34 (2017): 2675–83, https://doi.org/10.1089/neu.2016.4767; Steven Rowson et al., "Accounting for Variance in Concussion Tolerance between Individuals: Comparing Head Accelerations between Concussed and Physically Matched Control Subjects," *Annals of Biomedical Engineering* 47, no. 10 (2019): 2048–56, https://doi.org/10.1007/s10439-019-02329-7; Wilcox et al., "Head Impact Exposure."
72. Beckwith et al., "Timing of Concussion Diagnosis"; Brian D. Stemper et al., "Comparison of Head Impact Exposure between Concussed Football Athletes and Matched Controls: Evidence for a Possible Second Mechanism of Sport-Related Concussion," *Annals of Biomedical Engineering* 47, no. 10 (2018): 2057–72, https://doi.org/10.1007/s10439-018-02136-6.
73. Broglio et al., "Head Impact Density"; Stemper et al., "Comparison of Head Impact Exposure."

7. WHY HEAD IMPACTS IN YOUTH SPORTS MAY BE DISRUPTING BRAIN DEVELOPMENT

1. Alex Raskin, "NFL Legend Brett Favre Would Rather Be Remembered for ENDING Youth Tackle Football Than His Hall of Fame Career If It Means Saving Kids from the Head Traumas He Endured for Decades," *Daily Mail*, June 20, 2018, https://www.dailymail.co.uk/news/article-5866131/Brett-Favre-remembered-ENDING-youth-tackle-football-Hall-Fame-career.html.
2. Nowinski, "Youth Tackle Football."
3. Montenigro et al., "Cumulative Head Impact Exposure."
4. Julie M. Stamm et al., "Age of First Exposure to Football and Later-Life Cognitive Impairment in Former NFL Players," *Neurology* 84, no. 11 (2015): 1114–20, https://doi.org/10.1212/WNL.0000000000001358.
5. Julie M. Stamm et al., "Age at First Exposure to Football Is Associated with Altered Corpus Callosum White Matter Microstructure in Former Professional Football Players," *Journal of Neurotrauma* 32 (2015): 1768–76, https://doi.org/10.1089/neu.2014.3822.
6. Vivian Schultz et al., "Age at First Exposure to Repetitive Head Impacts Is Associated with Smaller Thalamic Volumes in Former Professional American Football Players," *Journal of Neurotrauma* 35, no. 2 (2017): 278–85, https://doi.org/10.1089/neu.2017.5145.
7. Timothy T. Brown et al., "Neuroanatomical Assessment of Biological Maturity," *Current Biology* 22, no. 18 (2012): 1693–98, https://doi.org/10.1016/j.cub.2012.07.002.
8. Gary S. Solomon et al., "Participation in Pre–High School Football and Neurological, Neuroradiological, and Neuropsychological Findings in Later Life: A Study of 45 Retired National Football League Players," *American Journal of Sports Medicine* 44, no. 5 (2016): 1106–15, https://doi.org/10.1177/0363546515626164.

9. M. L. Alosco et al., "Age of First Exposure to American Football and Long-Term Neuropsychiatric and Cognitive Outcomes," *Translational Psychiatry* 7, no. 9 (2017): e1236, https://doi.org/10.1038/tp.2017.197.

10. Andrea L. Roberts et al., "Exposure to American Football and Neuropsychiatric Health in Former National Football League Players: Findings from the Football Players Health Study," *American Journal of Sports Medicine* 47, no. 12 (2019): 2871–80, https://doi.org/10.1177/0363546519868989.

11. Barry R. Bryant et al., "The Effect of Age of First Exposure to Competitive Fighting on Cognitive and Other Neuropsychiatric Symptoms and Brain Volume," *International Review of Psychiatry* 32, no. 1 (2020): 89–95, https://doi.org/10.1080/09540261.2019.1665501.

12. Benjamin L. Brett et al., "Age of First Exposure to American Football and Behavioral, Cognitive, Psychological, and Physical Outcomes in High School and Collegiate Football Players," *Sports Health* 11, no. 4 (2019): 332–42, https://doi.org/10.1177/1941738119849076; Jaclyn B. Caccese et al., "Estimated Age of First Exposure to American Football and Neurocognitive Performance amongst NCAA Male Student-Athletes: A Cohort Study," *Sports Medicine* 49 (2019): 477–87, https://doi.org/10.1007/s40279-019-01069-x; Jaclyn B. Caccese et al., "Estimated Age of First Exposure to Contact Sports and Neurocognitive, Psychological, and Physical Outcomes in Healthy NCAA Collegiate Athletes: A Cohort Study," *Sports Medicine* 50, no. 7 (2020): 1377–92, https://doi.org/10.1007/s40279-020-01261-4; Jaclyn B. Caccese et al., "Estimated Age of First Exposure to Contact Sports Is Not Associated with Greater Symptoms or Worse Cognitive Functioning in Male U.S. Service Academy Athletes," *Journal of Neurotrauma* 37, no. 2 (2020): 334–39, https://doi.org/10.1089/neu.2019.6571.

13. Philip Schatz and Natalie Sandel, "Sensitivity and Specificity of the Online Version of ImPACT in High School and Collegiate Athletes," *American Journal of Sports Medicine* 41, no. 2 (2013): 321–26, https://doi.org/10.1177/0363546512466038.

14. Tracey Covassin et al., "Immediate Post-Concussion Assessment and Cognitive Testing (ImPACT) Practices of Sports Medicine Professionals," *Journal of Athletic Training* 44, no. 6 (2009): 639–44, https://doi.org/10.4085/1062-6050-44.6.639.

15. Timothy C. Durazzo et al., "Smoking and Increased Alzheimer's Disease Risk: A Review of Potential Mechanisms," *Alzheimer's & Dementia* 10, no. 3 (2014): S122–45, https://doi.org/10.1016/j.jalz.2014.04.009; Matthias Guggenmos et al., "Quantitative Neurobiological Evidence for Accelerated Brain Aging in Alcohol Dependence," *Translational Psychiatry* 7 (2017): 1279, https://doi.org/10.1038/s41398-017-0037-y; Adolf Pfefferbaum et al., "Accelerated Aging of Selective Brain Structures in HIV Infection: A Controlled, Longitudinal MRI Study," *Neurobiology of Aging* 35, no. 7 (2014): 1755–68, https://doi.org/10.1016/j.neurobiolaging.2014.01.008; Ilse Schuitema et al., "Accelerated Aging, Decreased White Matter Integrity, and Associated Neuropsychological Dysfunction 25 Years after Pediatric Lymphoid Malignancies," *Journal of Clinical Oncology* 31, no. 27 (2013): 3378–88, https://doi.org/10.1200/JCO.2012.46.7050.

8. WHY CTE IS MORE THAN AN NFL PROBLEM, AND WHAT IT MEANS FOR YOUTH SPORTS

1. Jeremy Allingham, "Brain Trust: Big Questions Surround the Most Influential Concussion Research on the Planet," *CBC News*, March 2, 2020, https://newsinteractives.cbc.ca/longform/brain-trust.

2. Ann C. McKee et al., "Chronic Traumatic Encephalopathy in Athletes: Progressive Tauopathy after Repetitive Head Injury," *Journal of Neuropathology and Experimental Neurology* 68, no. 7 (2009): 709–35, https://doi.org/10.1097/NEN.0b013e3181a9d503.

3. Harrison S. Martland, "Punch Drunk," *JAMA* 91 (1928): 1103–7.

4. K. M. Bowman and A. Blau, "Psychotic States following Head and Brain Injury in Adults and Children," in *Injuries of the Skull, Brain and Spinal Cord: Neuro-psychiatric, Surgical, and Medico-legal Aspects*, ed. S. Brock, 309–60 (Baltimore: Williams & Wilkins, 1940), https://doi.org/10.1037/11479-013.

5. National Collegiate Athletic Association, "Prevention and Care of Athletic Injuries: Recommendations for Medical Examination Pre-season Conditioning, Methods of Training, Diagnosis and Treatment of Injuries," in *National Collegiate Athletic Association Medical Handbook for Schools and Colleges* (Princeton, NJ: NCAA, 1933), 30–35.

6. Bennet I. Omalu et al., "Chronic Traumatic Encephalopathy in a National Football League Player," *Neurosurgery* 57, no. 1 (2005): 128–34, https://doi.org/10.1227/01.neu.0000163407.92769.ed.

7. Ann C. McKee et al., "The Spectrum of Disease in Chronic Traumatic Encephalopathy," *Brain* 136 (2013): 43–64, https://doi.org/10.1093/brain/aws307.

8. Miranda E. Orr, A. Campbell Sullivan, and Bess Frost, "A Brief Overview of Tauopathy: Causes, Consequences, and Therapeutic Strategies," *Trends in Pharmacological Sciences* 38, no. 7 (2017): 637–48, https://doi.org/10.1016/j.tips.2017.03.011.

9. McKee et al., "Spectrum of Disease."

10. McKee et al. "Spectrum of Disease."

11. R. J. H. Cloots et al., "Biomechanics of Traumatic Brain Injury: Influences of the Morphologic Heterogeneities of the Cerebral Cortex," *Annals of Biomedical Engineering* 36, no. 7 (2008): 203–15, https://doi.org/10.1007/s10439-008-9510-3.

12. Chad A. Tagge et al., "Concussion, Microvascular Injury, and Early Tauopathy in Young Athletes after Impact Head Injury and an Impact Concussion Mouse Model," *Brain* 141, no. 2 (2018): 422–58, https://doi.org/10.1093/brain/awx350.

13. Ann C. McKee et al., "The First NINDS/NIBIB Consensus Meeting to Define Neuropathological Criteria for the Diagnosis of Chronic Traumatic Encephalopathy," *Acta Neuropathologica* 131, no. 1 (2016): 75–86, https://doi.org/10.1007/s00401-015-1515-z.

14. McKee et al., "Spectrum of Disease."

15. Mez et al., "Clinicopathological Evaluation of Chronic Traumatic Encephalopathy"; Robert A. Stern et al., "Clinical Presentation of Chronic Traumatic Encephalopathy," *Neurology* 81 (2013): 1122–29, https://doi.org/10.1212/WNL.0b013e3182a55f7f.

16. Steven T. Dekosky and Kenneth Marek, "Looking Backward to Move Forward: Early Detection of Neurodegenerative Disorders," *Science* 302, no. 5646 (2003): 830–34, https://doi.org/10.1126/science.1090349.

17. Mez et al., "Clinicopathological Evaluation of Chronic Traumatic Encephalopathy"; Stern et al., "Clinical Presentation of Chronic Traumatic Encephalopathy."

18. Robert A. Stern et al., "Tau Positron-Emission Tomography in Former National Football League Players," *New England Journal of Medicine* 380, no. 18 (2019): 1716–25, https://doi.org/10.1056/NEJMoa1900757.

19. Michael L. Alosco et al., "Repetitive Head Impact Exposure and Later-Life Plasma Total Tau in Former National Football League Players," *Alzheimer's & Dementia: Diagnosis, Assessment & Disease Monitoring* 7 (2017): 33–40, https://doi.org/10.1016/j.dadm.2016.11.003; Michael L. Alosco et al., "Cerebrospinal Fluid Tau, Aβ, and sTREM2 in Former National Football League Players: Modeling the Relationship between Repetitive Head Impacts, Microglial Activation, and Neurodegeneration," *Alzheimer's & Dementia* 14, no. 9 (2018): 1159–70, https://doi.org/10.1016/j.jalz.2018.05.004.

20. Stern et al., "Tau Positron-Emission Tomography."

21. Gary W. Small et al., "PET Scanning of Brain Tau in Retired National Football League Players: Preliminary Findings," *American Journal of Geriatric Psychiatry* 21, no. 2 (2013): 138–44, https://doi.org/10.1016/j.jagp.2012.11.019.

22. Stern et al., "Tau Positron-Emission Tomography."

23. Mez et al., "Clinicopathological Evaluation of Chronic Traumatic Encephalopathy."

24. Zachary O. Binney and Kathleen E. Bachynski, "Estimating the Prevalence at Death of CTE Neuropathology among Professional Football Players," *Neurology* 92, no. 1 (2019): 43–45, https://doi.org/10.1212/WNL.0000000000006699.

25. Kevin A. Matthews et al., "Racial and Ethnic Estimates of Alzheimer's Disease and Related Dementias in the United States (2015–2060) in Adults Aged ≥65 Years," *Alzheimer's & Dementia* 15, no. 1 (2019): 17–24, https://doi.org/10.1016/j.jalz.2018.06.3063.

26. Adam M. Finkel and Kevin F. Bieniek, "A Quantitative Risk Assessment for Chronic Traumatic Encephalopathy (CTE) in Football: How Public Health Science Evaluates Evidence," *Human and Ecological Risk Assessment* 25, no. 3 (2019): 564–89, https://doi.org/10.1080/10807039.2018.1456899.

27. Everett J. Lehman et al., "Neurodegenerative Causes of Death among Retired National Football League Players," *Neurology* 79, no. 19 (2012): 1970–74, https://doi.org/10.1212/WNL.0b013e31826daf50; Daniel F. Mackay et al., "Neurodegenerative Disease Mortality among Former Professional Soccer Players," *New England Journal of Medicine* 381, no. 19 (2019): 1801–8, https://doi.org/10.1056/NEJMoa1908483; Vy T. Nguyen et al., "Mortality among Professional American-Style Football Players and Professional American Baseball Players," *JAMA Network Open* 2, no. 5 (2019): e194223, https://doi.org/10.1001/jamanetworkopen.2019.4223; Elisabetta Pupillo et al., "Increased Risk and Early Onset of ALS in Professional Players from Italian Soccer Teams," *Amyotrophic Lateral Sclerosis and Frontotemporal Dementia* 21, no. 5–6 (2020): 403–9, https://doi.org/10.1080/21678421.2020.1752250.

28. Jesse Mez et al., "Duration of American Football Play and Chronic Traumatic Encephalopathy," *Annals of Neurology* 87, no. 1 (2020): 116–31, https://doi.org/10.1002/ana.25611.

29. Mez et al. "Duration of American Football Play"; Mez et al., "Clinicopathological Evaluation of Chronic Traumatic Encephalopathy."

30. Kevin F. Bieniek et al., "Association between Contact Sports Participation and Chronic Traumatic Encephalopathy: A Retrospective Cohort Study," *Brain Pathology* 30, no. 1 (2019): 63–74, https://doi.org/10.1111/bpa.12757; Grant L. Iverson et al., "Mild Chronic Traumatic Encephalopathy Neuropathology in People with No Known Participation in Contact Sports or History of Repetitive Neurotrauma," *Journal of Neuropathology and Experimental Neurology* 78, no. 7 (2019): 615–25, https://doi.org/10.1093/jnen/nlz045.

31. Mez et al., "Duration of American Football Play."

32. Michael E. Buckland et al., "Chronic Traumatic Encephalopathy in Two Former Australian National Rugby League Players," *Acta Neuropathologica Communications* 7, no. 1 (2019): 97, https://doi.org/10.1186/s40478-019-0751-1; Edward B. Lee et al., "Chronic Traumatic Encephalopathy Is a Common Co-morbidity, but Less Frequent Primary Dementia in Former Soccer and Rugby Players," *Acta Neuropathologica* 138 (2019): 389–99, https://doi.org/10.1007/s00401-019-02030-y; McKee et al., "Chronic Traumatic Encephalopathy in Athletes"; McKee et al., "Spectrum of Disease"; Alan J. Pearce et al., "Chronic Traumatic Encephalopathy in a Former Australian Rules Football Player Diagnosed with Alzheimer's Disease," *Acta Neuropathologica Communications* 8 (2020): 23, https://doi.org/10.1186/s40478-020-0895-z; Alyssa Roenigk, "Doc-

tors Say Late BMX Legend Dave Mirra Had CTE," ESPN, May 24, 2016, https://www.espn.com/action/story/_/id/15614274/bmx-legend-dave-mirra-diagnosed-cte.

33. Lee E. Goldstein et al., "Chronic Traumatic Encephalopathy in Blast-Exposed Military Veterans and a Blast Neurotrauma Mouse Model," *Science Translational Medicine* 4, no. 134 (2012): 134ra60, https://doi.org/10.1126/scitranslmed.3003716; G. W. Roberts et al., "Dementia in a Punch-Drunk Wife," *Lancet* 335, no. 8694 (1990): 918–19, https://doi.org/10.1016/0140-6736(90)90520-f.

34. Mez et al., "Duration of American Football Play."

35. Thor D. Stein, Victor E. Alvarez, and Ann C. McKee, "Concussion in Chronic Traumatic Encephalopathy," *Current Pain and Headache Reports* 19, no. 10 (2015): 47, https://doi.org/10.1007/s11916-015-0522-z.

36. Ann C. McKee et al., "The Neuropathology of Sport," *Acta Neuropathologica* 127 (2014): 29–51, https://dx.doi.org/10.1007%2Fs00401-013-1230-6.

37. Bieniek et al., "Association between Contact Sports Participation"; McKee et al., "Chronic Traumatic Encephalopathy in Athletes."

38. "History of Title IX," Women's Sports Foundation, August 3, 2019, https://www.womenssportsfoundation.org/advocacy/history-of-title-ix/.

39. Christine M. Baugh et al., "Football Players' Perceptions of Future Risk of Concussion and Concussion-Related Health Outcomes," *Journal of Neurotrauma* 34 (2017): 790–97, https://doi.org/10.1089/neu.2016.4585.

40. Mez et al., "Duration of American Football Play."

41. Michael L. Alosco et al., "Age of First Exposure to Tackle Football and Chronic Traumatic Encephalopathy," *Annals of Neurology* 83 (2018): 886–901, https://doi.org/10.1002/ana.25245.

42. Mez et al., "Duration of American Football Play."

43. Durazzo et al., "Smoking and Increased Alzheimer's Disease Risk"; Guggenmos et al., "Quantitative Neurobiological Evidence"; Pfefferbaum et al., "Accelerated Aging of Selective Brain Structures."

44. Stern et al., "Clinical Presentation of Chronic Traumatic Encephalopathy."

45. Michael L. Alosco et al., "Cognitive Reserve as a Modifier of Clinical Expression in Chronic Traumatic Encephalopathy: A Preliminary Examination," *Journal of Neuropsychiatry and Clinical Neurosciences* 29, no. 1 (2017): 6–12, https://doi.org/10.1176/appi.neuropsych.16030043.

46. Finkel and Bieniek, "Quantitative Risk Assessment for Chronic Traumatic Encephalopathy."

9. WHY THE ARGUMENT THAT "OTHER SPORTS ARE DANGEROUS TOO" IS A BAD ONE

1. Maxwell Strachan, "Concussion Experts Pick Apart the Myth That Cycling Is More Dangerous Than Football," *Huffington Post*, March 20, 2015, https://www.huffpost.com/entry/football-biking-bicycling-nfl_n_6909714.

2. Aspen Institute, "2019 State of Play."

3. Kelly Sarmiento et al., "Emergency Department Visits for Sports- and Recreation-Related Traumatic Brain Injuries among Children—United States, 2010–2016," *Centers for Disease Control Morbidity and Mortality Weekly Report* 68, no. 10 (2019): 237–42, https://doi.org/10.15585/mmwr.mm6810a2.

4. Kerr et al., "Concussion Rates in U.S. Middle School Athletes"; Kerr et al., "Concussion Incidence and Trends in 20 High School Sports"; O'Kane et al., "Concussion among Female Middle-School Soccer Players."

5. Michael S. Schallmo, Joseph A. Weiner, and Wellington K. Hsu, "Sport and Sex-Specific Reporting Trends in the Epidemiology of Concussions Sustained by High School Athletes," *Journal of Bone and Joint Surgery American* 99, no. 15 (2017): 1314–20, https://doi.org/10.2106/JBJS.16.01573.

6. Jadischke et al., "Quantitative and Qualitative Analysis of Head and Body Impacts"; Lynall et al., "Comparison of Youth Flag and Tackle Football."

7. Andrew R. Peterson et al., "Youth Football Injuries: A Prospective Cohort," *Orthopaedic Journal of Sports Medicine* 5, no. 2 (2017), https://doi.org/10.1177/2325967116686784.

8. Kerr et al., "Concussion Rates in U.S. Middle School Athletes."

10. WHY HELMETS AND OTHER TECHNOLOGY WON'T SOLVE THE PROBLEM

1. "The End Zone," *The Documentary*, BBC Sounds, January 27, 2018, https://www.bbc.co.uk/sounds/play/w3cswdks.

2. Kathleen E. Bachynski and Daniel S. Goldberg, "Youth Sports and Public Health: Framing Risks of Mild Traumatic Brain Injury in American Football and Ice Hockey," *Journal of Law, Medicine, and Ethics* 42, no. 3 (2014): 323–33, https://doi.org/10.1111/jlme.12149.

3. Kathleen E. Bachynski and James M. Smoliga, "Pseudomedicine for Sports Concussions in the USA," *Lancet Neurology* S1474-4422, no. 19 (2019): 30250–59, https://doi.org/10.1016/S1474-4422(19)30250-9.

4. Shameemah Abrahams et al., "Risk Factors for Sports Concussion: An Evidence-Based Systematic Review," *British Journal of Sports Medicine* 48 (2014): 91–97, https://doi.org/10.1136/bjsports-2013-092734.

5. Erik E. Swartz et al., "A Helmetless-Tackling Intervention in American Football for Decreasing Head Impact Exposure: A Randomized Controlled Trial," *Journal of Science and Medicine in Sport* 22, no. 10 (2019): 1102–7, https://doi.org/10.1016/j.jsams.2019.05.018.

6. Michael L. Levy et al., "Birth and Evolution of the Football Helmet," *Neurosurgery* 55, no. 3 (2004): 656–62, https://doi.org/10.1227/01.NEU.0000134599.01917.AA.

7. J. Nadine Gelberg, "The Lethal Weapon: How the Plastic Football Helmet Transformed the Game of Football, 1939–1994," *Bulletin of Science, Technology, & Society* 15, no. 5–6 (1995): 302–9, https://doi.org/10.1177/0270467695015005-612.

8. Joseph J. Crisco and Richard M. Greenwald, "Let's Get the Head Further Out of the Game: A Proposal for Reducing Brain Injuries in Helmeted Contact Sports," *Current Sports Medicine Reports* 10, no. 1 (2011): 19–21.

9. Kathleen E. Bachynski, "'The Duty of Their Elders'—Doctors, Coaches, and the Framing of Youth Football's Health Risks, 1950s 1960s," *Journal of the History of Medicine and Allied Sciences* 74, no. 2 (2019): 167–91, https://doi.org/10.1093/jhmas/jry042.

10. Levy et al., "Birth and Evolution of the Football Helmet."

11. T. E., "Helmets, Game Speed and the Shifts That Dramatically Changed the NHL," *SB Nation*, March 21, 2012, https://www.sbnation.com/nhl/2012/3/21/2884609/nhl-helmet-usage-study-history.

12. Lukan, "Evolution of the Goalie Mask."

13. R. B. Fallstrom, "Last of Helmetless Players Retires," Associated Press, April 29, 1997, https://apnews.com/14215382dd33fe5113933e9298086782.

14. G. Van Rossem, "The Ninth Olympiad: Being the Official Report of the Olympic Games of 1928 Celebrated at Amsterdam" (Amsterdam, 1928), https://digital.la84.org/digital/collection/p17103coll8/id/13501.

15. Jon Mettus, "How Cascade Makes and Tests Helmets, Headgear," *USLacrosse Magazine*, January 19, 2017, https://www.uslaxmagazine.com/pro/industry/how-cascade-makes-and-tests-helmets-headgear.

16. Karen Given, "The Controversial History of Headgear in Girls' Lacrosse," WBUR, May 10, 2019, https://www.wbur.org/onlyagame/2019/05/10/girls-lacrosse-helmet-headgear-eyewear.

17. Crisco and Greenwald, "Let's Get the Head Further Out."

18. National Operating Committee on Standards for Athletic Equipment, "History," https://nocsae.org/about-nocsae/history/, accessed June 14, 2020.

19. ASTM International, "The History of ASTM International," https://www.astm.org/ABOUT/history_book.html, accessed June 14, 2020.

20. Crisco and Greenwald, "Let's Get the Head Further Out."

21. Matt Higgins, "Football Physics: The Anatomy of a Hit," *Popular Mechanics*, December 18, 2009, https://www.popularmechanics.com/adventure/sports/a2954/4212171/.

22. Sabrina Shankman, "Report Warned Riddell about Helmets," ESPN, April 30, 2013, https://www.espn.com/espn/otl/story/_/id/9228260/report-warned-riddell-no-helmet-prevent-concussions-nfl-helmet-maker-marketed-one-such-anyway.

23. Steven Rowson et al., "Can Helmet Design Reduce the Risk of Concussion in Football?," *Journal of Neurosurgery* 120 (2014): 919–22, https://doi.org/10.3171/2014.1.JNS13916.

24. Christy L. Collins et al., "Concussion Characteristics in High School Football by Helmet Age/Recondition Status, Manufacturer, and Model: 2008–2009 through 2012–2013 Academic Years in the United States," *American Journal of Sports Medicine* 44, no. 6 (2016): 1382–90, https://doi.org/10.1177/0363546516629626; Timothy A. McGuine et al., "Protective Equipment and Player Characteristics Associated with the Incidence of Sport-Related Concussion in High School Football Players: A Multifactorial Prospective Study," *American Journal of Sports Medicine* 42, no. 10 (2014): 2470–78, https://doi.org/10.1177/0363546514541926.

25. Micky Collins et al., "Examining Concussion Rates and Return to Play in High School Football Players Wearing Newer Helmet Technology: A Three-Year Prospective Cohort Study," *Neurosurgery* 58, no. 2 (2006): 257–86, https://doi.org/10.1227/01.NEU.0000200441.92742.46; Shankman, "Helmets."

26. Shankman, "Report Warned Riddell."

27. "Reebok-CCM Told It Can't Claim Hockey Helmet Protects against Concussion," CBC News, December 21, 2015, https://www.cbc.ca/news/business/hockey-helmet-concussions-1.3375030.

28. "Virginia Tech Helmet Ratings," https://helmet.beam.vt.edu/index.html, accessed June 14, 2020.

29. Caccese and Kaminski, "Minimizing Head Acceleration"; Cam Smith, "Virginia Tech Helmet Lab Releases New Youth Football Helmet Ratings; Seven Models Receive Top Grades," *USA Today*, March 22, 2019, https://usatodayhss.com/2019/virginia-tech-helmet-lab-releases-new-youth-football-helmet-ratings-seven-models-receive-top-grades.

30. Katherine M. Breedlove et al., "The Ability of an Aftermarket Helmet Add-On Device to Reduce Impact-Force Accelerations during Drop Tests," *Journal of Athletic Training* 52, no. 9 (2017): 802–8, https://doi.org/10.4085/1062-6050-52.6.01.

31. J. S. Delaney et al., "The Effect of Protective Headgear on Head Injuries and Concussions in Adolescent Football (Soccer) Players," *British Journal of Sports Medicine* 42, no. 2 (2008): 110–15, https://doi.org/10.1136/bjsm.2007.037689.

32. Timothy McGuine et al., "Does Soccer Headgear Reduce the Incidence of Sport-Related Concussion? A Cluster, Randomised Controlled Trial of Adolescent Athletes," *British Journal of Sports Medicine* 54, no. 7 (2020): 408–13, https://doi.org/10.1136/bjsports-2018-100238.

33. Stephanie J. Hollis et al., "Incidence, Risk, and Protective Factors of Mild Traumatic Brain Injury in a Cohort of Australian Nonprofessional Male Rugby Players," *American Journal of Sports Medicine* 37, no. 12 (2009): 2328–33, https://doi.org/10.1177/0363546509341032; Simon P. T. Kemp et al., "The Epidemiology of Head Injuries in English Professional Rugby Union," *Clinical Journal of Sport Medicine* 18, no. 3 (2008): 227–34, https://doi.org/10.1097/JSM.0b013e31816a1c9a.

34. Andrew S. Mcintosh et al., "Does Padded Headgear Prevent Head Injury in Rugby Union Football?," *Medicine & Science in Sports & Exercise* 41, no. 2 (2009): 306–13, https://doi.org/10.1249/MSS.0b013e3181864bee.

35. Abrahams et al., "Risk Factors for Sports Concussion"; Brian W. Benson et al., "What Are the Most Effective Risk-Reduction Strategies in Sport Concussion?," *British Journal of Sports Medicine* 47 (2013): 321–26, https://doi.org/10.1136/bjsports-2013-092216.

36. McGuine et al., "Protective Equipment."

37. O'Connor et al., "Head-Impact–Measurement Devices."

38. Beckwith et al., "Head Impact Exposure"; Broglio, Lapointe, and Connor, "Head Impact Density"; Rowson et al., "Accounting for Variance."

39. O'Connor et al., "Head-Impact–Measurement Devices."

40. Bachynski and Smoliga, "Pseudomedicine for Sports Concussions."

41. Mike Freeman, "Russell Wilson Sending a Dangerous Message with Supposed Miracle Concussion Cure," *Bleacher Report*, August 28, 2015, https://bleacherreport.com/articles/2555884-russell-wilson-sending-a-dangerous-message-with-supposed-miracle-concussion-cure.

42. Bachynski and Smoliga, "Pseudomedicine for Sports Concussions."

43. Gregory D. Myer et al., "The Effects of External Jugular Compression Applied during Head Impact Exposure on Longitudinal Changes in Brain Neuroanatomical and Neurophysiological Biomarkers: A Preliminary Investigation," *Frontiers in Neurology* 7 (2016): 74, https://doi.org/10.3389/fneur.2016.00074.

44. George Farah, Donald Siwek, and Peter Cummings, "Tau Accumulations in the Brains of Woodpeckers," *PLOS ONE* 13, no. 2 (2018): e0191526, https://doi.org/10.1371/journal.pone.0191526.

45. Christy L. Collins et al., "Neck Strength: A Protective Factor Reducing Risk for Concussion in High School Sports," *Journal of Primary Prevention* 35, no. 5 (2014): 309–19, https://doi.org/10.1007/s10935-014-0355-2; Zachary D. W. Dezman, Eric H. Ledet, and Hamish A. Kerr, "Neck Strength Imbalance Correlates with Increased Head Acceleration in Soccer Heading," *Sports Health* 5, no. 4 (2013): 320–26, https://doi.org/10.1177/1941738113480935.

46. Stephan Becker et al., "Effects of a 6-Week Strength Training of the Neck Flexors and Extensors on the Head Acceleration during Headers in Soccer," *Journal of Sports Science & Medicine* 18, no. 4 (2019): 729–37; Mihalik et al., "Does Cervical Muscle Strength"; Julianne D. Schmidt et al., "The Influence of Cervical Muscle Characteristics on Head Impact Biomechanics in Football," *American Journal of Sports Medicine* 42, no. 9 (2014): 2056–66, https://doi.org/10.1177/0363546514536685.

47. Collins et al., "Neck Strength."

11. WHY "SAFER THAN EVER" MAY NOT BE SAFE ENOUGH

1. Jason Galloway, "The Concussion Question: NCAA Concussion, Head Trauma Messaging Remains Work in Progress," *Wisconsin State Journal*, August 14, 2018, https://madison.com/wsj/news/local/health-med-fit/the-concussion-question-ncaa-concussion-head-trauma-messaging-remains-work/article_1148189e-cb79-5184-8817-e0fb4428f3f1.html.

2. Tom Farrey and Jon Solomon, "What If . . . Flag Becomes the Standard Way of Playing Football until High School? An Aspen Institute Sports & Society Program Analysis," 2018, https://assets.aspeninstitute.org/content/uploads/2018/09/FINAL-Future-of-Football-Paper.4.pdf?_ga=2.50021478.1369729969.1554144622-1005435048.1554144622.

3. Belson, "To Allay Fears, N.F.L. Huddles with Mothers"; Mike Florio, "NFL Pushes Back on Youth Football 'Myths,'" *Pro Football Talk NBC Sports*, May 8, 2019, https://profootballtalk.nbcsports.com/2019/05/08/nfl-pushes-back-on-youth-football-myths/.

4. Bachynski, "'Duty of Their Elders'"; Jim Weathersby, "Teddy Roosevelt's Role in the Creation of the NCAA," *Sports Historian*, July 6, 2016, https://www.thesportshistorian.com/teddy-roosevelts-role-in-the-creation-of-the-ncaa/.

5. National Center for Catastrophic Sport Injury Research, "Reports," https://nccsir.unc.edu/reports/, accessed June 23, 2020.

6. National Center for Catastrophic Sport Injury Research, "Reports."

7. James Craig Brown et al., "The Incidence of Rugby-Related Catastrophic Injuries (Including Cardiac Events) in South Africa from 2008 to 2011: A Cohort Study," *BMJ Open* 3, no. 2 (2013): e002475, https://doi.org/10.1136/bmjopen-2012-002475; Collin W. Fuller, "Catastrophic Injury in Rugby Union: Is the Level of Risk Acceptable?," *Sports Medicine* 38, no. 12 (2008): 975–86, https://doi.org/10.2165/00007256-200838120-00002.

8. Brian D. Stemper et al., "Repetitive Head Impact Exposure in College Football following an NCAA Rule Change to Eliminate Two-a-Day Preseason Practices: A Study from the NCAA-DoD CARE Consortium," *Annals of Biomedical Engineering* 47, no. 10 (2019): 2073–85, https://doi.org/10.1007/s10439-019-02335-9.

9. Brian D. Stemper et al., "Head Impact Exposure in College Football following a Reduction in Preseason Practices," *Medicine & Science in Sports & Exercise* 52, no. 7 (2020): 1629–38, https://doi.org/10.1249/MSS.0000000000002283.

10. USA Hockey, "Standard of Play and Rule Emphasis—Body Checking," https://www.usahockeyrulebook.com/page/show/1015119-standard-of-play-and-rule-emphasis-body-checking#, accessed June 23, 2020.

11. Carolyn A. Emery et al., "Risk of Injury Associated with Body Checking among Youth Ice Hockey Players," *JAMA* 303, no. 22 (2010): 2265–72, https://doi.org/10.1001/jama.2010.755.

12. Black et al., "Risk of Injury Associated with Body Checking."

13. Amanda M. Black et al., "Policy Change Eliminating Body Checking in Non-elite Ice Hockey Leads to a Threefold Reduction in Injury and Concussion Risk in 11- and 12-Year-Old Players," *British Journal of Sports Medicine* 50 (2016): 55–61, https://doi.org/10.1136/bjsports-2015-095103; Black et al., "Risk of Injury Associated with Body Checking"; Emery et al., "Risk of Injury Associated with Body Checking"; Carolyn Emery et al., "Does Disallowing Body Checking in Non-elite 13- to 14-Year-Old Ice

Hockey Leagues Reduce Rates of Injury and Concussion? A Cohort Study in Two Canadian Provinces," *British Journal of Sports Medicine* 54, no. 7 (2019): 414–20, https://doi.org/10.1136/bjsports-2019-101092.

14. David P. Trofa et al., "The Impact of Body Checking on Youth Ice Hockey Injuries," *Orthopaedic Journal of Sports Medicine* 5, no. 12 (2015): 1–4, https://doi.org/10.1177/2325967117741647.

15. USA Hockey, "Hockey in the United States."

16. Black et al., "Risk of Injury Associated with Body Checking."

17. Emery et al., "Risk of Injury Associated with Body Checking."

18. Richard Hinton, "Youth Lacrosse Participation," MedStar Sports Medicine, https://www.medstarsportsmedicine.org/about-us/partnership-with-us-lacrosse/youth-lacrosse-participation/, accessed June 20, 2020.

19. US Lacrosse, "Boys' Youth Rules Book, 2020," https://www.uslacrosse.org/sites/default/files/public/documents/rules/YouthRulebook-Boys2020-spreads.pdf.

20. Kerr et al., "Injury Incidence in Youth, High School, and NCAA Men's Lacrosse."

21. Sebastian Salazar, "U.S. Soccer Bans Headers for Children under Age 10," *NBC Sports*, November 12, 2015, https://www.nbcsports.com/washington/soccer/us-soccer-bans-headers-children-under-age-10.

22. US Youth Soccer, "US Youth Soccer Policy on Players and Playing Rules," February 16, 2019, http://www.usyouthsoccer.org/assets/56/6/us_youth_soccer_policy_on_players_and_playing_rules.pdf.

23. "FA Guidelines: Children to No Longer Head Footballs during Training," *BBC News*, February 24, 2020, https://www.bbc.com/news/uk-scotland-51614088; Nayanah Siva, "Scotland to Ban Heading in Children's Football," *Lancet* 395, no. 10220 (2020): 258, https://doi.org/10.1016/S0140-6736(20)30118-5.

24. Vince Rugari, "'Watching These Kids Head a Ball Was Crazy': FFA to Review Heading Policy," *Sydney Morning Herald*, February 26, 2020, https://www.smh.com.au/sport/soccer/watching-these-kids-head-a-ball-was-crazy-ffa-to-review-heading-policy-20200226-p544h2.html.

25. Frederic Gilbert and Bradely J. Partridge, "The Need to Tackle Concussion in Australian Football Codes," *Medical Journal of Australia* 196, no. 9 (2012): 561–63, https://doi.org/10.5694/mja11.11218.

26. Keith A. Stokes et al., "Does Reducing the Height of the Tackle through Law Change in Elite Men's Rugby Union (The Championship, England) Reduce the Incidence of Concussion? A Controlled Study in 126 Games," *British Journal of Sports Medicine* (2019): 1–6, https://doi.org/10.1136/bjsports-2019-101557.

27. Chad Wise, "Contact in Youth Rugby," USA Rugby, March 13, 2014, https://www.usa.rugby/2014/03/contact-in-youth-rugby/; Rugby AU, "Laws Summary for U6-U12," 2020, https://australia.rugby/participate/referee/laws; NRL Touch Football, "Welcome to Touch Football," https://touchfootball.com.au/, accessed June 17, 2020.

28. USA Rugby, "USA Rugby Eagle Roadmap," 2018, https://assets.usa.rugby/docs/eagles-roadmap.pdf.

29. Bachynski, "'Duty of Their Elders.'"

30. Douglas J. Wiebe et al., "Association between the Experimental Kickoff Rule and Concussion Rates in Ivy League Football," *JAMA* 320, no. 19 (2018): 2035–36, https://doi.org/10.1001/jama.2018.14165.

31. Adam Y. Pfaller et al., "Effect of a New Rule Limiting Full Contact Practice on the Incidence of Sport-Related Concussion in High School Football Players," *American Journal of Sports Medicine* 47, no. 10 (2019): 2294–99, https://doi.org/10.1177/0363546519860120.

32. Mark Maske, "Concussions Were Down This Past Season on NFL Kickoffs," *Washington Post*, March 1, 2019, https://www.washingtonpost.com/sports/2019/03/01/concussions-were-down-this-past-season-nfl-kickoffs/?noredirect=on.

33. USA Football, "Rookie Tackle," 2020, https://usafootball.com/rookietackle/.

34. USA Football, "Football Development Model: How the Model Works," 2020, https://fdm.usafootball.com/how-it-works.

35. Zachary Y. Kerr et al., "Comprehensive Coach Education and Practice Contact Restriction Guidelines Result in Lower Injury Rates in Youth American Football," *Orthopaedic Journal of Sports Medicine* 3, no. 7 (2015): 1–8, https://doi.org/10.1177/2325967115594578.

36. Alan Schwarz, "N.F.L.-Backed Youth Program Says It Reduced Concussions. The Data Disagrees," *New York Times*, July 27, 2016, https://www.nytimes.com/2016/07/28/sports/football/nfl-concussions-youth-program-heads-up-football.html.

37. Galloway, "Concussion Question."

38. Steve Fainaru and Mark Fainaru-Wada, "Questions about Heads Up Tackling," ESPN, January 10, 2014, https://www.espn.com/espn/otl/story/_/id/10276129/popular-nfl-backed-heads-tackling-method-questioned-former-players.

39. Schwarz, "N.F.L.-Backed Youth Program."

40. Kerr et al., "Comprehensive Coach Education and Practice."

41. Zachary Y. Kerr et al., "Comprehensive Coach Education Reduces Head Impact Exposure in American Youth Football," *Orthopaedic Journal of Sports Medicine* 3, no. 10 (2015): 1–6, https://doi.org/10.1177/2325967115610545.

42. Robert F. Heary, Neil Majmundar, and Roxanne Nagurka, "Is Youth Football Safe? An Analysis of Youth Football Head Impact Data," *Neurosurgery* 87, no. 2 (2020): 377–82, https://doi.org/10.1093/neuros/nyz563.

43. Bachynski, "'Duty of Their Elders.'"

44. Swartz et al., "Helmetless-Tackling Intervention."

45. Larry Lage, "AP Survey: Most States Limit Full Contact for HS Football," Associated Press, August 30, 2019, https://apnews.com/e525659c28734de98da719a110893d21.

46. Pfaller et al., "Effect of a New Rule."

47. Cobb et al., "Head Impact Exposure in Youth Football."

48. Broglio et al., "Football Players' Head-Impact Exposure."

49. Broglio et al., "Football Players' Head-Impact Exposure."

50. Cobb et al., "Head Impact Exposure in Youth Football."

51. Montenigro et al., "Cumulative Head Impact Exposure."

52. Hosea Harvey and Policy Surveillance Program Staff, "Youth Sports Traumatic Brain Injury Laws," Policy Surveillance Program, June 30, 2017, https://lawatlas.org/datasets/sc-reboot.

53. Stamm et al., "Awareness of Concussion Education Requirements."

54. Mark Beakey et al., "Is It Time to Give Athletes a Voice in the Dissemination Strategies of Concussion-Related Information? Exploratory Examination of 2444 Adolescent Athletes," *Clinical Journal of Sport Medicine* 30, no. 6 (2020): 562–67, https://doi.org/10.1097/JSM.0000000000000653.

55. Register-Mihalik et al., "Demographic, Parental, and Personal Factors"; Sarmiento, Donnell, and Hoffman, "Scooping Review to Address the Culture of Concussion"; Wallace, Covassin, and Beidler, "Sex Differences in High School Athletes' Knowledge."

56. Kearney and See, "Misunderstandings of Concussion"; Stamm et al., "Awareness of Concussion Education Requirements."

57. Kerr et al., "Motivations Associated with Non-disclosure"; Sarmiento, Donnell, and Hoffman, "Scooping Review to Address the Culture of Concussion."

58. Sara P. D. Chrisman et al., "Parents' Perspectives regarding Age Restrictions for Tackling in Youth Football," *Pediatrics* 143, no. 5 (2019): e20182402, https://doi.org/10.1542/peds.2018-2402.

59. Schallmo, Weiner, and Hsu, "Sport and Sex-Specific Reporting Trends."

60. Ryan Swanson, "Why the Latest Effort to Make Youth Football Safer Could Fail," *Washington Post*, August 23, 2019, https://www.washingtonpost.com/outlook/2019/08/23/why-latest-effort-make-youth-football-safer-could-fail/?noredirect=on.

12. WHY YOU DON'T HAVE TO HIT AT A YOUNG AGE TO BE A SUPERSTAR

1. David Schuman, "'You Can Play Flag Football': Romo on Board with Favre Comments to Stop Tackling in Youth Football," WDJT Milwaukee, June 21, 2018, https://www.cbs58.com/news/you-can-play-flag-football-romo-on-board-with-favre-comments-to-stop-tackling-in-youth-football.

2. Derek Thompson, "American Meritocracy Is Killing Youth Sports," *Atlantic*, November 6, 2018, https://www.theatlantic.com/ideas/archive/2018/11/income-inequality-explains-decline-youth-sports/574975/.

3. Concussion Legacy Foundation, "Flag Football Under 14: All Time Greatest Team," 2018, https://concussionfoundation.org/programs/flag-football/all-time-team.

4. "Michael Strahan," Vibe, https://www.vibe.com/p/michael-strahan, accessed May 30, 2020.

5. Jerome Bettis, "Story of My Life," *Players' Tribune*, September 22, 2016, https://www.theplayerstribune.com/en-us/articles/jerome-bettis-story-of-my-life.

6. "Rugby Late Starters and Bloomers," Where to Play Rugby, April 30, 2019, https://wheretoplayrugby.com/news/2019/04/30/rugby-late-starters-and-bloomers/.

7. USA Rugby, "The Official Website of USA Rugby," http://usa.rugby/, accessed June 10, 2020.

8. USA Rugby, "Alev Kelter," https://www.usa.rugby/player/alev-kelter/, accessed June 10, 2020.

9. Tom Farrey, "Miracle on Ice," ESPN, June 26, 2013, https://www.espn.com/nhl/story/_/id/9418183/usa-hockey-encourages-kids-nhl-dreams-play-other-sports-espn-magazine.

10. USA Hockey, "Hockey in the United States."

11. Farrey and Solomon, "What If . . ."

12. NCAA, "Estimated Probability of Competing in College Athletics."

13. NCAA, "Estimated Probability of Competing in Professional Athletics," 2020, http://www.ncaa.org/about/resources/research/estimated-probability-competing-professional-athletics.

14. Ashley J. Cripps, Luke S. Hopper, and Christopher Joyce, "Can Coaches Predict Long-Term Career Attainment Outcomes in Adolescent Athletes?," *International Journal of Sports Science and Coaching* 14, no. 3 (2019): 324–28, https://doi.org/10.1177/1747954119848418.

15. Carolyn Emery et al., "Risk of Injury Associated with Bodychecking Experience among Youth Hockey Players," *CMAJ* 183, no. 11 (2011): 1249–56, https://doi.org/10.1503/cmaj.110634; Alison Macpherson, Linda Rothman, and Andrew Howard, "Body-Checking Rules and Childhood Injuries in Ice Hockey," *Pediatrics* 117, no. 2 (2006): e143–47, https://doi.org/10.1542/peds.2005-1163; Trofa et al., "Impact of Body Checking."

16. Macpherson, Rothman, and Howard, "Body-Checking Rules."

17. Pfaller et al., "Effect of a New Rule."

18. Rhodri S. Lloyd et al., "National Strength and Conditioning Association Position Statement on Long-Term Athletic Development," *Journal of Strength and Conditioning Research* 30, no. 6 (2016): 1491–1509, https://doi.org/10.1519/JSC.000000000000 1387.

19. David R. Bell et al., "Sport Specialization and Risk of Overuse Injuries: A Systematic Review with Meta-Analysis," *Pediatrics* 142, no. 3 (2018): e20180657, https://doi.org/10.1542/peds.2018-0657.

20. Lloyd et al., "National Strength and Conditioning Association Position."

21. Ben Cohen, "Jim Harbaugh's Advice to Football Recruits: Play Soccer," *Wall Street Journal*, August 14, 2017, https://www.wsj.com/articles/jim-harbaughs-advice-to-football-recruits-play-soccer-1502729321?mod=e2fb.

13. WHY THE BENEFITS OF SPORTS CAN BE GAINED WITHOUT REPETITIVE BRAIN TRAUMA

1. Robert M. Malina et al., "Overweight and Obesity among Youth Participants in American Football," *Journal of Pediatrics* 151, no. 4 (2007): 378–82, https://doi.org/10.1016/j.jpeds.2007.03.044.

2. Bachynski, "'Duty of Their Elders.'"

3. Camiré and Trudel, "Using High School Football."

4. Roger Pielke Jr., "Has the United States Reached Peak (American) Football?," Play the Game, September 25, 2017, https://www.playthegame.org/news/comments/2017/048_has-the-united-states-reached-peak-american-football/.

5. David W. Brown et al., "Adverse Childhood Experiences and the Risk of Premature Mortality," *American Journal of Preventive Medicine* 37, no. 5 (2009): 389–96, https://doi.org/10.1016/j.amepre.2009.06.021.

6. Brody et al., "Protective Prevention Effects"; McLaughlin, Weissman, and Bitrán, "Childhood Adversity."

7. de Greeff et al., "Effects of Physical Activity on Executive Functions"; Eime et al., "Systematic Review."

8. Molly C. Easterlin et al., "Association of Team Sports Participation with Long-Term Mental Health Outcomes among Individuals Exposed to Adverse Childhood Experiences," *JAMA Pediatrics* 173, no. 7 (2019): 681–88, https://doi.org/10.1001/jamapediatrics.2019.1212.

9. Allyson M. Pollock and Graham Kirkwood, "Removing Contact from School Rugby Will Not Turn Children into Couch Potatoes," *British Journal of Sports Medicine* 50, no. 16 (2016): 963–64, https://doi.org/10.1136/bjsports-2016-096220.

10. Danny M. Pincivero and Tudor O. Bompa, "A Physiological Review of American Football," *Sports Medicine* 23, no. 4 (1997): 247–60, https://doi.org/10.2165/00007256-199723040-00004.

11. Michael Kanters et al., "Physical Activity Report," Healthy Sport Index, 2018, https://healthysportindex.com/report/physical-activity/.

12. Ken Belson, "The N.F.L.'s Obesity Scourge," *New York Times*, January 17, 2019, https://www.nytimes.com/2019/01/17/sports/football/the-nfls-obesity-scourge.html.

13. Jackie L. Buell et al., "Presence of Metabolic Syndrome in Football Linemen," *Journal of Athletic Training* 43, no. 6 (2008): 608–16, https://doi.org/10.4085/1062-6050-43.6.608.

14. Belson, "N.F.L.'s Obesity Scourge."

15. Belson, "N.F.L.'s Obesity Scourge."

16. Tyler Maas, "Remembering (and Re-experiencing) Burger King's 'Gilbertburger,'" *Milwaukee Record*, November 9, 2018, https://milwaukeerecord.com/sports/remembering-and-re-experiencing-burger-kings-gilbertburger/.

17. J. Steinberger et al., "Comparison of Body Fatness Measurements by BMI and Skinfolds vs Dual Energy X-Ray Absorptiometry and Their Relation to Cardiovascular Risk Factors in Adolescents," *International Journal of Obesity* 29, no. 11 (2005): 1346–52, https://doi.org/10.1038/sj.ijo.0803026.

18. Kelly R. Laurson and Joey C. Eisenmann, "Prevalence of Overweight among High School Football Linemen," *JAMA* 297, no. 4 (2007): 363–64, https://doi.org/10.1001/jama.297.4.363.

19. Laurson and Eisenmann, "Prevalence of Overweight"; Asheley Cockrell Skinner et al., "Is Bigger Really Better? Obesity among High School Football Players, Player Position, and Team Success," *Clinical Pediatrics* 52, no. 10 (2013): 922–28, https://doi.org/10.1177/0009922813492880.

20. Skinner et al., "Is Bigger Really Better?"

21. Malina et al., "Overweight and Obesity."

14. HOW WE CAN CHANGE CONTACT SPORTS TO PROTECT CHILDREN'S BRAINS

1. Mike Florio, "John Madden Doesn't Believe in the Heads Up Football Program," *Pro Football Talk*, NBC Sports, August 5, 2014, https://profootballtalk.nbcsports.com/2014/08/05/john-madden-doesnt-believe-in-the-heads-up-football-program/.

2. Jim Morrison, "The Early History of Football's Forward Pass," *Smithsonian Magazine*, December 28, 2010, https://www.smithsonianmag.com/history/the-early-history-of-footballs-forward-pass-78015237/.

3. NFL Football Operations, "Bent but Not Broken: The History of the Rules," https://operations.nfl.com/the-rules/evolution-of-the-nfl-rules/, accessed June 13, 2020.

4. T. E., "Helmets, Game Speed and the Shifts."

5. USA Hockey, "Hockey in the United States."

6. Lewis Steele, "How the Back-Pass Rule Changed Football in England Almost Overnight," *These Football Times*, October 17, 2018, https://thesefootballtimes.co/2018/10/17/how-the-back-pass-rule-changed-football-in-england-almost-overnight/.

7. Farrey and Solomon, "What If . . ."

8. NFHS, "High School Sports Participation Increases for 29th Consecutive Year," September 11, 2018, https://www.nfhs.org/articles/high-school-sports-participation-increases-for-29th-consecutive-year; NFHS, "Participation in High School Sports Registers First Decline in 30 Years," September 5, 2019, https://www.nfhs.org/articles/participation-in-high-school-sports-registers-first-decline-in-30-years/.

9. Ken Belson et al., "Inside Football's Campaign to Save the Game," *New York Times*, November 7, 2019, https://www.nytimes.com/interactive/2019/11/08/sports/falling-football-participation-in-america.html.

10. Bob Cook, "Why High School Football Is Dying a Slow Death (It's Not Just Concussions)," *Forbes*, August 31, 2018, https://www.forbes.com/sites/bobcook/2018/

08/31/why-high-school-football-is-dying-a-slow-death-its-not-just-concussions/ #5d079be87540.

11. Joshua J. Dyck, Francis T. Talty, and Jeffrey Gerson, "Citizen Attitudes about Sports, Concussions and CTE May 31–June 6, 2016," 2016, https://www.uml.edu/docs/ cpor-concussion-highlights_tcm18-248453.pdf.

12. Barrow Neurological Institute, "Barrow Concussion Survey."

13. Chrisman et al., "Parents' Perspectives."

14. Shpigel, "Luke Kuechly."

15. Steve Fainaru and Mark Fainaru-Wada, "For the NFL and All of Football, a New Threat: An Evaporating Insurance Market," ESPN, January 17, 2019.

16. Steven H. Miles and Shailendra Prasad, "Medical Ethics and School Football," *American Journal of Bioethics* 16, no. 1 (2016): 6–10, https://doi.org/10.1080/ 15265161.2016.1128751.

17. Roger Piekle, "The Decline of Football Is Real and It's Accelerating," *Forbes*, January 28, 2020, https://www.forbes.com/sites/rogerpielke/2020/01/28/the-decline-of-football-is-real-and-its-accelerating/#7d5cf88e2f37.

18. Farrey and Solomon, "What If . . ."

19. Aspen Institute, "2019 State of Play."

20. Barrow Neurological Institute, "Barrow Concussion Survey."

21. NFHS, "Participation in High School Sports Registers First Decline."

22. Dyck, Talty, and Gerson, "Citizen Attitudes."

23. Black et al., "Policy Change Eliminating Body Checking"; Emery et al., "Risk of Injury Associated with Body Checking."

24. USA Hockey, "Hockey in the United States."

25. Council on Sports Medicine and Fitness et al., "Reducing Injury Risk from Body Checking in Boys' Youth Ice Hockey," *Pediatrics* 133, no. 6 (2014): 1151–57, https:// doi.org/10.1542/peds.2014-0692.

26. Emery et al., "Does Disallowing Body Checking."

27. Black et al., "Risk of Injury Associated with Body Checking."

28. Taylor A. Lee et al., "Distribution of Head Acceleration Events Varies by Position and Play Type in North American Football," *Clinical Journal of Sport Medicine* (2020), https://doi.org/10.1097/JSM.0000000000000778.

29. Pop Warner Little Scholars, "Pop Warner Becomes First National Football Organization to Eliminate 3-Point Stance," February 28, 2019, https://www.popwarner. com/Default.aspx?tabid=1403205&mid=1475016&newskeyid=HN1&newsid= 279263&ctl=newsdetail.

30. Jon Solomon, "American Heritage Football's Limited-Contact Practices Have Led to Championships," *USA Today*, September 11, 2019, https://usatodayhss.com/ 2019/american-heritage-football-limited-contact-practices-aspen-institute-award.

31. Roman Stubbs, "This High School Football Team Never Tackled in Practice Last Year. Then It Won a State Title," *Washington Post*, August 27, 2019, https://www. washingtonpost.com/sports/2019/08/27/this-high-school-football-team-never-tackled-practice-last-year-then-it-won-state-title/.

32. Marc Tracy, "The Ivy League Becomes the Future of Football," *New York Times*, October 26, 2018, https://www.nytimes.com/2018/10/26/sports/ivy-league-football-dartmouth.html.

33. Saint John's University Johnnies, "John Gagliardi," https://gojohnnies.com/staff-directory/john-gagliardi/9, accessed June 20, 2020.

34. Pfaller et al., "Effect of a New Rule."

35. Beckwith et al., "Head Impact Exposure"; Stemper et al., "Comparison of Head Impact Exposure."

36. National Flex Football, https://www.flexfootball.com/, accessed June 20, 2020.

37. Joseph Toninato et al., "Injury Rate in TackleBar Football," *Orthopaedic Journal of Sports Medicine* 7, no. 10 (2019), https://doi.org/10.1177/2325967119874065.

38. Concussion Legacy Foundation, "Flag Football Under 14," https://concussionfoundation.org/programs/flag-football, accessed June 20, 2020.

39. Austin Danforth, "Is Flag Football or Tackle Football the Future for Vermont Youth Leagues? Debate Simmers," *Burlington Free Press*, September 5, 2018, https://www.burlingtonfreepress.com/story/sports/high-school/football/2018/09/05/vermont-high-school-football-flag-football-future-youths/1056532002/.

40. Pfaller et al., "Effect of a New Rule."

41. Concussion Legacy Foundation, "Flag Football Under 14."

42. Football 'N' America, https://www.playfna.com/, accessed June 20, 2020.

43. Council on Sports Medicine and Fitness et al., "Reducing Injury Risk from Body Checking"; Council on Sports Medicine and Fitness, "Tackling in Youth Football," *Pediatrics* 136, no. 5 (2015): e1419–30, https://doi.org/10.1542/peds.2015-3282.

44. Lerner and Fost, "Informed Consent."

45. Mark Dunphy, "Here's What Happened in the Five Other States That Tried to Ban Youth Tackle Football," Boston.com, March 3, 2019, https://www.boston.com/sports/parenting/2019/03/03/massachusetts-proposed-law-ban-youth-tackle-football.

46. Jake Niall and Peter Ryan, "Call to End 'Warrior Culture' after CTE Discovered in AFL Legend's Brain," *Age*, February 27, 2020, https://www.theage.com.au/sport/afl/call-to-end-the-warrior-culture-after-cte-discovered-in-afl-legend-s-brain-20200227-p5454k.html.

47. Allyson M. Pollock, Adam John White, and Graham Kirkwood, "Evidence in Support of the Call to Ban the Tackle and Harmful Contact in School Rugby: A Response to World Rugby," *British Journal of Sports Medicine* 51 (2017): 1113–17, https://doi.org/10.1136/bjsports-2016-096996.

48. Mihalik et al., "Effect of Infraction Type."

49. Kuriyama, Nakatsuka, and Yamamoto, "High School Football Players Use Their Helmets."

50. Stokes et al., "Does Reducing the Height."

51. Jon Solomon, "American Heritage Football's Limited-Contact Practices Have Led to Championships," *USA Today*, September 11, 2017, https://usatodayhss.com/2019/american-heritage-football-limited-contact-practices-aspen-institute-award.

52. Lerner and Fost, "Informed Consent."

53. Miles and Prasad, "Medical Ethics."

54. Dee Warmath and Andrew P. Winterstein, "A Social-Marketing Intervention and Concussion-Reporting Beliefs," *Journal of Athletic Training* 55, no. 10 (2020): 1035–45, https://doi.org/10.4085/1062-6050-242-19.

55. Emily Kroshus and Sara P. D. Chrisman, "A New Game Plan for Concussion Education," *Health Education & Behavior* 46, no. 6 (2019): 916–21, https://doi.org/10.1177/1090198119859414.

56. Kroshus et al., "Threat, Pressure, and Communication."

57. Baugh et al., "Perceived Coach Support."

58. Beakey et al., "Is It Time to Give Athletes."

59. Emily Kroshus, Zachary Y. Kerr, and Joseph G. L. Lee, "Community-Level Inequalities in Concussion Education of Youth Football Coaches," *American Journal of Preventive Medicine* 52, no. 4 (2017): 476–82, https://doi.org/10.1016/j.amepre.2016.12.021.

60. Robbins et al., "Self-Reported Concussion History"; Alissa Wicklund, Ashley Roy, and J. Douglas Coatsworth, "Providing a Medical Definition of Concussion: Can a Simple Intervention Improve Self-Reported Concussion History in Youth Athletes?," *Clinical Journal of Sport Medicine* (2020), https://doi.org/10.1097/JSM.0000000000000813.

61. Dee Warmath and Andrew P. Winterstein, "Reporting Skill: The Missing Ingredient in Concussion Reporting Intention Assessment," *Sports Health* 1, no. 5 (2019): 416–24, https://doi.org/10.1177/1941738119856609.

62. Kroshus and Chrisman, "New Game Plan."

63. E. Kroshus et al., "Talking with Young Children about Concussions: An Exploratory Study," *Child: Care, Health, and Development* 43, no. 5 (2017): 758–67, https://doi.org/10.1111/cch.12433.

64. Nancy Armour, "Opinion: Fighting in the NHL Is Brutish and Outdated, and Needs to Be Banned," *USA Today*, April 16, 2019, https://www.usatoday.com/story/sports/columnist/nancy-armour/2019/04/16/nhl-playoffs-no-reason-league-should-continue-allowing-fighting/3490209002/.

65. Mihalik et al., "Effect of Infraction Type."

66. Mihalik et al., "Effect of Infraction Type."

67. Aynsley M. Smith et al., "Behavioral Modification to Reduce Concussion in Collision Sports: Ice Hockey," *Current Sports Medicine Reports* 12, no. 6 (2013): 3–6, https://doi.org/10.1249/JSR.0000000000000004.

68. Schmidt et al., "Safe-Play Knowledge"; Smith et al., "Behavioral Modification."

69. Guo Chen Liew et al., "Mental Toughness in Sport: Systematic Review and Future," *German Journal of Exercise and Sport Research* 49 (2019): 381–94, https://doi.org/10.1007/s12662-019-00603-3.

15. WHAT FAMILIES AND ATHLETES CAN DO TO STAY SAFE IN YOUTH SPORTS

1. Kathleen E. Bachynski, "Youth Football Is a Moral Abdication," *Atlantic*, February 1, 2020, https://www.theatlantic.com/ideas/archive/2020/02/youth-football-moral-abdication/605932/.

2. John O. Spengler, "Getting and Keeping Kids in the Game: A Summary of Key Recommendations by Medical and Health Groups," Aspen Institute, 2014.

3. Bell et al., "Sport Specialization."

4. National Athletic Trainers Association, "Proper Fit = Proper Protection," https://www.nata.org/sites/default/files/football-helmet-handout.pdf, accessed April 5, 2020.

5. Centers for Disease Control and Prevention, "What Is a Concussion?"

6. Karlin, "Concussion in the Pediatric and Adolescent Population"; Kroshus et al., "Talking with Young Children."

7. Aneetinder Mann, Charles H. Tator, and James D. Carson, "Concussion Diagnosis and Management: Knowledge and Attitudes of Family Medicine Residents," *Canadian Family Physician* 63 (2017): 460–66.

16. WHAT YOU CAN DO TO IMPROVE THE SAFETY OF YOUTH SPORTS IN YOUR COMMUNITY

1. Aspen Institute, "2019 State of Play."

2. Aspen Institute, "2019 State of Play."

3. Timothy A. McGuine et al., "The Influence of Athletic Trainers on the Incidence and Management of Concussions in High School Athletes," *Journal of Athletic Training* 53, no. 11 (2018): 1017–24, https://doi.org/10.4085/1062-6050-209-18.

4. DeMatteo et al., "Effectiveness of Return to Activity."

5. Aspen Institute, "2019 State of Play."

6. Lloyd et al., "National Strength and Conditioning Association Position."

7. Maguire A. B. Herriman, "The Need for an Intervention to Prevent Sports Injuries beyond 'Rub Some Dirt on It,'" *JAMA Pediatrics* 173, no. 3 (2019): 215–16, https://doi.org/10.1001/jamapediatrics.2018.4602.

CONCLUSION

1. Alan Pearce, "Concern for Athletes Is Not Making Footy Soft," NeuroPearce, 2019, https://neuropearce.com/news#8f5915f5-a336-45e6-bbb7-31747b1450a8.

2. Jerome O. Nriagu, "Clair Patterson and Robert Kehoe's Paradigm of 'Show Me the Data' on Environmental Lead Poisoning," *Environmental Research* 78 (1998): 71–78, https://doi.org/10.1006/enrs.1997.3808.

3. Malcom Gladwell, "Burden of Proof," *Revisionist History* podcast, 2018, http://revisionisthistory.com/episodes/22-burden-of-proof.

4. Bachynski, "'Duty of Their Elders.'"

5. Lerner and Fost, "Informed Consent."

Selected Bibliography

Ackerman, Sandra. *Discovering the Brain*. Washington DC: National Academies Press (US), 1992. https://www.ncbi.nlm.nih.gov/books/NBK234146/.

Alosco, M. L., A. B. Kasimis, J. M. Stamm, A. S. Chua, C. M. Baugh, D. H. Daneshvar, C. A. Robbins, et al. "Age of First Exposure to American Football and Long-Term Neuropsychiatric and Cognitive Outcomes." *Translational Psychiatry* 7, no. 9 (2017): e1236. https://doi.org/10.1038/tp.2017.197.

Alosco, Michael L., Jesse Mez, Yorghos Tripodis, Patrick T. Kiernan, Bobak Abdolmo- hammadi, Lauren Murphy, Neil W. Kowall, et al. "Age of First Exposure to Tackle Football and Chronic Traumatic Encephalopathy." *Annals of Neurology* 83 (2018): 886–901. https://doi.org/10.1002/ana.25245.

Andersen, Susan L., and Martin H. Teicher. "Stress, Sensitive Periods and Maturational Events in Adolescent Depression." *Trends in Neurosciences* 31, no. 4 (2008): 183–91. https://doi.org/10.1016/j.tins.2008.01.004.

Anderson, Vicki, Megan Spencer-Smith, and Amanda Wood. "Do Children Really Re- cover Better? Neurobehavioural Plasticity after Early Brain Insult." *Brain* 134, no. 8 (2011): 2197–2221. https://doi.org/10.1093/brain/awr103.

Aspen Institute. "2019 State of Play: Trends and Developments in Youth Sports." https://www.aspeninstitute.org/wp-content/uploads/2019/10/2019_SOP_National_Final.pdf.

Ayer, Julian, Marietta Charakida, John E. Deanfield, and David S. Celermajer. "Life- time Risk: Childhood Obesity and Cardiovascular Risk." *European Heart Journal* 36 (2015): 1371–76. https://doi.org/10.1093/eurheartj/ehv089.

Bachynski, Kathleen E. "'The Duty of Their Elders'—Doctors, Coaches, and the Fram- ing of Youth Football's Health Risks, 1950s–1960s." *Journal of the History of Medi- cine and Allied Sciences* 74, no. 2 (2019): 167–91. https://doi.org/10.1093/jhmas/jry042.

Bahrami, Naelm, Dev Sharma, Scott Rosenthal, Elizabeth M. Davenport, Jillian E. Urban, Benjamin Wagner, Youngkyoo Jung, et al. "Subconcussive Head Impact Exposure and White Matter Tract Changes over a Single Season of Youth Football." *Radiology* 281, no. 3 (2016): 919–26. https://doi.org/10.1148/radiol.2016160564.

Bari, Sumra, Diana O. Svaldi, Ikbeom Jang, Trey E. Shenk, Victoria N. Poole, Taylor Lee, Ulrike Dydak, et al. "Dependence on Subconcussive Impacts of Brain

Metabolism in Collision Sport Athletes: An MR Spectroscopic Study." *Brain Imaging and Behavior* 13, no. 3 (2019): 735–49. https://doi.org/10.1007/s11682-018-9861-9.

Barrow Neurological Institute. "Barrow Concussion Survey: Fewer Parents Let Kids Play Contact Sports." August 22, 2019. https://www.barrowneuro.org/press-releases/barrow-concussion-survey-fewer-parents-let-kids-play-contact-sports/.

Baugh, Christine M., Emily Kroshus, Patrick T. Kiernan, David Mendel, and William P. Meehan III. "Football Players' Perceptions of Future Risk of Concussion and Concussion-Related Health Outcomes." *Journal of Neurotrauma* 34 (2017): 790–97. https://doi.org/10.1089/neu.2016.4585.

Bazarian, Jeffrey J., Tong Zhu, Jianhui Zhong, Damir Janigro, Eric Rozen, Andrew Roberts, Hannah Javien, et al. "Persistent, Long-Term Cerebral White Matter Changes after Sports-Related Repetitive Head Impacts." *PLOS ONE* 9, no. 4 (2014): e94734. https://doi.org/10.1371/journal.pone.0094734.

Beckwith, Jonathan G., Richard M. Greenwald, Jeffrey J. Chu, Joseph J. Crisco, Steven Rowson, Stefan M. Duma, Steven P. Broglio, et al. "Head Impact Exposure Sustained by Football Players on Days of Diagnosed Concussion." *Medicine & Science in Sports & Exercise* 45, no. 4 (2013): 737–46. https://doi.org/10.1249/MSS.0b013e3182792ed7.

Beckwith, Jonathan G, Richard M Greenwald, Jeffrey J Chu, Joseph J Crisco, Steven Rowson, Stefan M. Duma, Steven P. Broglio, et al. "Timing of Concussion Diagnosis Is Related to Head Impact Exposure Prior to Injury." *Medicine & Science in Sports & Exercise* 45, no. 4 (2014): 747–54. https://doi.org/10.1249/MSS.0b013e3182793067.

Bellamkonda, Srinidhi, Samantha J. Woodward, Eamon Campolettano, Ryan Gellner, Mireille E. Kelley, Derek A. Jones, Amaris Genemaras, et al. "Head Impact Exposure in Practices Correlates with Exposure in Games for Youth Football Players." *Journal of Applied Biomechanics* 34, no. 5 (2018): 354–60. https://doi.org/10.1123/jab.2017-0207.

Bieniek, Kevin F., Melissa M. Blessing, Michael G. Heckman, Nancy N. Diehl, Amanda M. Serie, Michael A. Paolini, Bradley F. Boeve, et al. "Association between Contact Sports Participation and Chronic Traumatic Encephalopathy: A Retrospective Cohort Study." *Brain Pathology* 30, no. 1 (2019): 63–74. https://doi.org/10.1111/bpa.12757.

Black, Amanda M., Brent E. Hagel, Luz Palacios-Derflingher, Kathryn J. Schneider, and Carolyn A. Emery. "The Risk of Injury Associated with Body Checking among Pee Wee Ice Hockey Players: An Evaluation of Hockey Canada's National Body Checking Policy Change." *British Journal of Sports Medicine* 51 (2017): 1767–72. https://doi.org/10.1136/bjsports-2016-097392.

Black, Amanda M., Alison K. MacPherson, Brent E. Hagel, Maria A. Romiti, Luz Palacios-Derflingher, Jian Kang, Willem H. Meeuwisse, et al. "Policy Change Eliminating Body Checking in Non-elite Ice Hockey Leads to a Threefold Reduction in Injury and Concussion Risk in 11- and 12-Year-Old Players." *British Journal of Sports Medicine* 50 (2016): 55–61. https://doi.org/10.1136/bjsports-2015-095103.

Bohr, Adam D., Jason D. Boardman, and Matthew B. McQueen. "Association of Adolescent Sport Participation with Cognition and Depressive Symptoms in Early Adulthood." *Orthopaedic Journal of Sports Medicine* 7, no. 9 (2019): 1–11. https://doi.org/10.1177/2325967119868658.

Brett, Benjamin L., Daniel L. Huber, Alexa Wild, Lindsay D. Nelson, and Michael A. McCrea. "Age of First Exposure to American Football and Behavioral, Cognitive, Psychological, and Physical Outcomes in High School and Collegiate Football Players." *Sports Health* 11, no. 4 (2019): 332–42. https://doi.org/10.1177/1941738119849076.

Bretzin, Abigail C., Tracey Covassin, Meghan E. Fox, Kyle M. Petit, Jennifer L. Savage, Lauren F. Walker, and Daniel Gould. "Sex Differences in the Clinical Incidence of Concussions, Missed School Days, and Time Loss in High School Student-Athletes." *American Journal of Sports Medicine* 46, no. 9 (2018): 2263–69. https://doi.org/10.1177/0363546518778251.

Broglio, Steven P., James T. Eckner, Douglas Martini, Jacob J. Sosnoff, Jeffrey S. Kutcher, and Christopher Randolph. "Cumulative Head Impact Burden in High School Football." *Journal of Neurotrauma* 28 (2011): 2069–78. https://doi.org/10.1089/neu.2011.1825.

Broglio, Steven P., Andrew Lapointe, and Kathryn L. O'Connor. "Head Impact Density: A Model to Explain the Elusive Concussion Threshold." *Journal of Neurotrauma* 34 (2017): 2675–83. https://doi.org/10.1089/neu.2016.4767.

Broglio, Steven P., Douglas Martini, Luke Kasper, James T. Eckner, and Jeffrey S. Kutcher. "Estimation of Head Impact Exposure in High School Football: Implications for Regulating Contact Practices." *American Journal of Sports Medicine* 41, no. 12 (2013): 2877–84. https://doi.org/10.1177/0363546513502458.

Broglio, Steven P., Brock Schnebel, Jacob J. Sosnoff, Sunghoon Shin, Xingdong Feng, Xuming He, and Jerrad Zimmerman. "Biomechanical Properties of Concussions in High School Football." *Medicine & Science in Sports & Exercise* 42, no. 11 (2010): 2064–71. https://doi.org/10.1249/MSS.0b013e3181dd9156.

Broglio, Steven P., Richelle M. Williams, Kathryn L. O'Connor, and Jason Goldstick. "Football Players' Head-Impact Exposure after Limiting of Full-Contact Practices." *Journal of Athletic Training* 51, no. 7 (2016): 511–18. https://doi.org/10.4085/1062-6050-51.7.04.

Caccese, Jaclyn B., Barry A. Bodt, Grant L. Iverson, Thomas W. Kaminski, Kelsey Bryk, Jessie Oldham, Steven P. Broglio, et al. "Estimated Age of First Exposure to Contact Sports and Neurocognitive, Psychological, and Physical Outcomes in Healthy NCAA Collegiate Athletes: A Cohort Study." *Sports Medicine* 50, no. 7 (2020): 1377–92. https://doi.org/10.1007/s40279-020-01261-4.

Caccese, Jaclyn B., Ryan M. Dewolf, Thomas W. Kaminski, Steven P. Broglio, Thomas W. McAllister, Michael McCrea, Thomas A. Buckley, et al. "Estimated Age of First Exposure to American Football and Neurocognitive Performance amongst NCAA Male Student-Athletes: A Cohort Study." *Sports Medicine* 49 (2019): 477–87. https://doi.org/10.1007/s40279-019-01069-x.

Caccese, Jaclyn B., Grant L. Iverson, Kenneth L. Cameron, Megan N. Houston, Gerald McGinty, Jonathan C. Jackson, Patrick O'Donnell, et al. "Estimated Age of First Exposure to Contact Sports Is Not Associated with Greater Symptoms or Worse Cognitive Functioning in Male U.S. Service Academy Athletes." *Journal of Neurotrauma* 37, no. 2 (2020): 334–39. https://doi.org/10.1089/neu.2019.6571.

Cacucci, Francesca, and Faraneh Vargha-Khadem. "Contributions of Nonhuman Primate Research to Understanding the Consequences of Human Brain Injury during Development." *PNAS* 116, no. 52 (2019): 26204–9. https://doi.org/10.1073/pnas.1912952116.

Campolettano, Eamon T., Ryan A. Gellner, Eric P. Smith, Srinidhi Bellamkonda, Casey T. Tierney, Joseph J. Crisco, Derek A. Jones, et al. "Development of a Concussion Risk Function for a Youth Population Using Head Linear and Rotational Acceleration." *Annals of Biomedical Engineering* 48, no. 1 (2019): 92–103. https://doi.org/10.1007/s10439-019-02382-2.

Centers for Disease Control and Prevention. "What Is a Concussion?" Heads Up, February 12, 2019. https://www.cdc.gov/headsup/basics/concussion_whatis.html.

Champagne, Allen A., Nicole S. Coverdale, Mike Germuska, Alex A. Bhogal, and Douglas J. Cook. "Changes in Volumetric and Metabolic Parameters Relate to Differences in Exposure to Sub-concussive Head Impacts." *Journal of Cerebral Blood*

Flow & Metabolism 40, no. 7 (2020): 1453–67. https://doi.org/10.1177/0271678X19862861.

Chrisman, Sara P. D., Beth E. Ebel, Elizabeth Stein, Sarah J. Lowry, and Frederick P. Rivara. "Head Impact Exposure in Youth Soccer and Variation by Age and Sex." *Clinical Journal of Sport Medicine* 29, no. 1 (2019): 3–10. https://doi.org/10.1097/JSM.0000000000000497.

Chrisman, Sara P. D., Kathryn B. Whitlock, Emily Kroshus, Christina Schwien, Stanley A. Herring, and Frederick P. Rivara. "Parents' Perspectives regarding Age Restrictions for Tackling in Youth Football." *Pediatrics* 143, no. 5 (2019): e20182402. https://doi.org/10.1542/peds.2018-2402.

Churchill, Nathan W., Michael G. Hutchison, Simon J. Graham, and Tom A. Schweizer. "Mapping Brain Recovery after Concussion: From Acute Injury to 1 Year after Medical Clearance." *Neurology* 93, no. 21 (2019): e1980–92. https://doi.org/10.1212/WNL.0000000000008523.

Cobb, Bryan R., Jillian E. Urban, Elizabeth M. Davenport, Steven Rowson, Stefan M. Duma, Joseph A. Maldjian, Christopher T. Whitlow, et al. "Head Impact Exposure in Youth Football: Elementary School Ages 9–12 Years and the Effect of Practice Structure." *Annals of Biomedical Engineering* 41, no. 12 (2013): 2463–73. https://doi.org/10.1007/s10439-013-0867-6.

Collins, Micky, Mark R. Lovell, Grant L. Iverson, Thad Ide, and Joseph Maroon. "Examining Concussion Rates and Return to Play in High School Football Players Wearing Newer Helmet Technology: A Three-Year Prospective Cohort Study." *Neurosurgery* 58, no. 2 (2006): 257–86. https://doi.org/10.1227/01.NEU.0000200441.92742.46.

Concussion Legacy Foundation. "Flag Football Under 14." https://concussionfoundation.org/programs/flag-football. Accessed June 20, 2020.

Council on Sports Medicine and Fitness. "Tackling in Youth Football." *Pediatrics* 136, no. 5 (2015): e1419–30. https://doi.org/10.1542/peds.2015-3282.

Council on Sports Medicine and Fitness, Alison Brooks, Keith J. Loud, Joel S. Brenner, Rebecca A. Demorest, Mark E. Halstead, Amanda K. Weiss Kelly, et al. "Reducing Injury Risk from Body Checking in Boys' Youth Ice Hockey." *Pediatrics* 133, no. 6 (2014): 1151–57. https://doi.org/10.1542/peds.2014-0692.

Crews, Fulton, Jun He, and Clyde Hodge. "Adolescent Cortical Development: A Critical Period of Vulnerability for Addiction." *Pharmacology, Biochemistry and Behavior* 86, no. 2 (2007): 189–99. https://doi.org/10.1016/j.pbb.2006.12.001.

Crisco, Joseph J., and Richard M. Greenwald. "Let's Get the Head Further Out of the Game: A Proposal for Reducing Brain Injuries in Helmeted Contact Sports." *Current Sports Medicine Reports* 10, no. 1 (2011): 19–21.

Crisco, Joseph J., Bethany J. Wilcox, Jonathan G. Beckwith, Jeffrey J. Chu, Ann-Christine Duhaime, Steven Rowson, Stefan M. Duma, et al. "Head Impact Exposure in Collegiate Football Players." *Journal of Biomechanics* 44, no. 15 (2011): 2673–78. https://doi.org/10.1016/j.jbiomech.2011.08.003.

Crisco, Joseph J., Bethany J. Wilcox, Jason T. Machan, Thomas W. McAllister, Christine Duhaime, Stefan M. Duma, Steven Rowson, et al. "Magnitude of Head Impact Exposures in Individual Collegiate Football Players." *Journal of Applied Biomechanics* 28, no. 2 (2013): 174–83. https://doi.org/10.1123/jab.28.2.174.

Daniel, Ray W., Steven Rowson, and Stefan M. Duma. "Head Impact Exposure in Youth Football." *Annals of Biomedical Engineering* 40, no. 4 (2012): 976–81. https://doi.org/10.1007/s10439-012-0530-7.

Daniel, Ray W., Steven Rowson, and Stefan M. Duma. "Head Impact Exposure in Youth Football: Middle School Ages 12–14 Years." *Journal of Biomechanical Engineering* 136, no. 9 (2014): 094501. https://doi.org/10.1115/1.4027872.

Daniel, Thomas A., Kyle M. Townsend, Yun Wang, David S. Martin, Jeffrey S. Katz, and Gopikrishna Deshpande. "North American Football Fans Show Neurofunctional Differences in Response to Violence: Implications for Public Health and Policy." *Frontiers in Public Health* 6, no. July (2018): 1–9. https://doi.org/10.3389/fpubh.2018.00177.

Deshpande, Sameer K., Raiden B. Hasegawa, Amanda R. Rabinowitz, John Whyte, Carol L. Roan, Andrew Tabatabaei, Michael Baiocchi, et al. "Association of Playing High School Football with Cognition and Mental Health Later in Life." *JAMA Neurology* 74, no. 8 (2017): 909–18. https://doi.org/10.1001/jamaneurol.2017.1317.

Deshpande, Sameer K., Raiden B. Hasegawa, Jordan Weiss, and Dylan S. Small. "The Association between Adolescent Football Participation and Early Adulthood Depression." *PLOS ONE* 15, no. 3 (2020): e0229978. https://doi.org/10.1371/journal.pone.0229978.

Easterlin, Molly C., Paul J. Chung, Mei Leng, and Rebecca Dudovitz. "Association of Team Sports Participation with Long-Term Mental Health Outcomes among Individuals Exposed to Adverse Childhood Experiences." *JAMA Pediatrics* 173, no. 7 (2019): 681–88. https://doi.org/10.1001/jamapediatrics.2019.1212.

Eckner, James T., Kathryn L. O'Connor, Steven P. Broglio, and James A. Ashton-Miller. "Comparison of Head Impact Exposure between Male and Female High School Ice Hockey Athletes." *American Journal of Sports Medicine* 46, no. 9 (2018): 2253–62. https://doi.org/10.1177/0363546518777244.

Eime, Rochelle M., Janet A. Young, Jack T. Harvey, Melanie J. Charity, and Warren R. Payne. "A Systematic Review of the Psychological and Social Benefits of Participation in Sport for Children and Adolescents: Informing Development of a Conceptual Model of Health through Sport." *International Journal of Behavioral Nutrition and Physical Activity* 10, no. 98 (2013): 1–21. https://doi.org/10.1186/1479-5868-10-98.

Emery, Carolyn A., Jian Kang, Ian Shrier, Claude Goulet, Brent E. Hagel, Brian W. Benson, Alberto Nettel-Aguirre, et al. "Risk of Injury Associated with Body Checking among Youth Ice Hockey Players." *JAMA* 303, no. 22 (2010): 2265–72. https://doi.org/10.1001/jama.2010.755.

Emery, Carolyn, Jian Kang, Ian Shrier, Claude Goulet, Brent Hagel, Brian Benson, Alberto Nettel-Aguirre, et al. "Risk of Injury Associated with Bodychecking Experience among Youth Hockey Players." *CMAJ* 183, no. 11 (2011): 1249–56. https://doi.org/10.1503/cmaj.101540.

Emery, Carolyn, Luz Palacios-Derflingher, Amanda Marie Black, Paul Eliason, Maciek Krolikowski, Nicole Spencer, Stacy Kozak, et al. "Does Disallowing Body Checking in Non-elite 13- to 14-Year-Old Ice Hockey Leagues Reduce Rates of Injury and Concussion? A Cohort Study in Two Canadian Provinces." *British Journal of Sports Medicine* 54, no. 7 (2019): 414–20. https://doi.org/10.1136/bjsports-2019-101092.

Farrey, Tom, and Jon Solomon. "What If . . . Flag Becomes the Standard Way of Playing Football until High School? An Aspen Institute Sports & Society Program Analysis." 2018. https://assets.aspeninstitute.org/content/uploads/2018/09/FINAL-Future-of-Football-Paper.4.pdf?_ga=2.50021478.1369729969.1554144622-1005435048.1554144622.

Finkel, Adam M., and Kevin F. Bieniek. "A Quantitative Risk Assessment for Chronic Traumatic Encephalopathy (CTE) in Football: How Public Health Science Evaluates Evidence." *Human and Ecological Risk Assessment* 25, no. 3 (2019): 564–89. https://doi.org/10.1080/10807039.2018.1456899.

Giedd, Jay N., Jonathan Blumenthal, Neal O. Jeffries, F. X. Castellanos, Hong Liu, Alex Zijdenbos, Tomáš Paus, et al. "Brain Development during Childhood and Adolescence: A Longitudinal MRI Study." *Nature Neuroscience* 2, no. 10 (1999): 861–63. https://doi.org/10.1038/13158.

Guskiewicz, Kevin M., and Tamara C. Valovich McLeod. "Pediatric Sports-Related Concussion." *PM&R* 3, no. 4 (2011): 353–64. https://doi.org/10.1016/j.pmrj.2010. 12.006.

Hanlon, Erin M., and Cynthia A. Bir. "Real-Time Head Acceleration Measurement in Girls' Youth Soccer." *Medicine & Science in Sports & Exercise* 44, no. 6 (2012): 1102–8. https://doi.org/10.1249/MSS.0b013e3182444d7d.

Iverson, Grant L., Teemu M. Luoto, Pekka J. Karhunen, and Rudolph J. Castellani. "Mild Chronic Traumatic Encephalopathy Neuropathology in People with No Known Participation in Contact Sports or History of Repetitive Neurotrauma." *Journal of Neuropathology and Experimental Neurology* 78, no. 7 (2019): 615–25. https://doi.org/10.1093/jnen/nlz045.

Jadischke, Ron, Jessica Zendler, Erik Lovis, Andrew Elliott, and Grant C. Goulet. "Quantitative and Qualitative Analysis of Head and Body Impacts in American 7v7 Non-tackle Football." *BMJ Open Sport & Exercise Medicine* 6, no. 1 (2020): e000638. https://doi.org/10.1136/bmjsem-2019-000638.

Janda, David H., Cynthia A. Bir, and Angela L. Cheney. "An Evaluation of the Cumulative Concussive Effect of Soccer Heading in the Youth Population." *Injury Control and Safety Promotion* 9, no. 1 (2002): 25–31. https://doi.org/10.1076/icsp.9.1.25. 3324.

Jang, Ikbeom, Il Yong Chun, Jared R. Brosch, Sumra Bari, Yukai Zou, Brian R. Cummiskey, Taylor A. Lee, et al. "Every Hit Matters: White Matter Diffusivity Changes in High School Football Athletes Are Correlated with Repetitive Head Acceleration Event Exposure." *NeuroImage: Clinical* 24 (2019): 101930. https://doi.org/10.1016/j.nicl.2019.101930.

Karlin, Aaron M. "Concussion in the Pediatric and Adolescent Population: 'Different Population, Different Concerns.'" *PM&R* 3, no. 10 Suppl 2 (2011): S369–79. https://doi.org/10.1016/j.pmrj.2011.07.015.

Kerr, Zachary Y., Avinash Chandran, Aliza K. Nedimyer, Alan Arakkal, Lauren A. Pierpoint, and Scott L. Zuckerman. "Concussion Incidence and Trends in 20 High School Sports." *Pediatrics* 144, no. 5 (2019): e20192180. https://doi.org/10.1542/peds.2019-2180.

Kerr, Zachary Y., Nelson Cortes, Amanda M. Caswell, Jatin P. Ambegaonkar, Kaitlin Romm Hallsmith, A. Frederick Milbert, and Shane V. Caswell. "Concussion Rates in U.S. Middle School Athletes, 2015–2016 School Year." *American Journal of Preventive Medicine* 53, no. 6 (2017): 914–18. https://doi.org/10.1016/j.amepre.2017.05. 017.

Kerr, Zachary Y., Johna K. Register-Mihalik, Emily Kroshus, Christine M. Baugh, and Stephen W. Marshall. "Motivations Associated with Non-disclosure of Self-Reported Concussions in Former Collegiate Athletes." *American Journal of Sports Medicine* 44, no. 1 (2016): 220–25. https://doi.org/10.1177/0363546515612082.

Kerr, Zachary Y., Susan W. Yeargin, Tamara C. Valovich McLeod, James Mensch, Ross Hayden, and Thomas P. Dompier. "Comprehensive Coach Education Reduces Head Impact Exposure in American Youth Football." *Orthopaedic Journal of Sports Medicine* 3, no. 10 (2015): 1–6. https://doi.org/10.1177/2325967115610545.

Kerr, Zachary Y., Susan Yeargin, Tamara C. Valovich McLeod, Vincent C. Nittoli, James Mensch, Thomas Dodge, Ross Hayden, et al. "Comprehensive Coach Education and Practice Contact Restriction Guidelines Result in Lower Injury Rates in Youth American Football." *Orthopaedic Journal of Sports Medicine* 3, no. 7 (2015): 1–8. https://doi.org/10.1177/2325967115594578.

King, Doug, Patria Hume, Conor Gissane, and Trevor Clark. "Head Impacts in a Junior Rugby League Team Measured with a Wireless Head Impact Sensor: An Exploratory Analysis." *Journal of Neurosurgery: Pediatrics* 19 (2017): 13–23. https://doi.org/10. 3171/2016.7.PEDS1684.

King, Doug A., Patria A. Hume, Conor Gissane, and Trevor N. Clark. "Similar Head Impact Acceleration Measured Using Instrumented Ear Patches in a Junior Rugby Union Team during Matches in Comparison with Other Sports." *Journal of Neurosurgery: Pediatrics* 18 (2016): 65–72. https://doi.org/10.3171/2015.12.PEDS15605.

Koerte, Inga K., Birgit Ertl-Wagner, Maximilian Reiser, Ross Zafonte, and Martha E. Shenton. "White Matter Integrity in the Brains of Professional Soccer Players without a Symptomatic Concussion." *JAMA* 308, no. 18 (2012): 1859–61. https://doi.org/10.1001/jama.2012.13735.

Koerte, Inga K., Michael Mayinger, Marc Muehlmann, David Kaufmann, Alexander P. Lin, Denise Steffinger, Barbara Fisch, et al. "Cortical Thinning in Former Professional Soccer Players." *Brain Imaging and Behavior* 10 (2016): 792–98. https://doi.org/10.1007/s11682-015-9442-0.

Koerte, Inga K., Elizabeth Nichols, Yorghos Tripodis, Vivian Schultz, Stefan Lehner, Randy Igbinoba, Alice Z. Chuang, et al. "Impaired Cognitive Performance in Youth Athletes Exposed to Repetitive Head Impacts." *Journal of Neurotrauma* 34 (2017): 2389–95. https://doi.org/10.1089/neu.2016.4960.

Kroshus, Emily, Christine M. Baugh, Cynthia J. Stein, S. Bryn Austin, and Jerel P. Calzo. "Concussion Reporting, Sex, and Conformity to Traditional Gender Norms in Young Adults." *Journal of Adolescence* 54 (2017): 110–19. https://doi.org/10.1016/j.adolescence.2016.11.002.

Kroshus, Emily, Bernice Garnett, Matt Hawrilenko, Christine M. Baugh, and Jerel P. Calzo. "Concussion Under-Reporting and Pressure from Coaches, Teammates, Fans, and Parents." *Social Science and Medicine* 134 (2015): 66–75. https://doi.org/10.1016/j.socscimed.2015.04.011.

Kuriyama, Andrew M., Austin S. Nakatsuka, and Loren G. Yamamoto. "High School Football Players Use Their Helmets to Tackle Other Players Despite Knowing the Risks." *Hawai'i Journal of Medicine & Public Health* 76, no. 3 (2017): 77–81.

Lamond, Lindsey C., Jaclyn B. Caccese, Thomas A. Buckley, Joseph Glutting, and Thomas W. Kaminski. "Linear Acceleration in Direct Head Contact across Impact Type, Player Position, and Playing Scenario in Collegiate Women's Soccer Players." *Journal of Athletic Training* 53, no. 2 (2018): 115–21. https://doi.org/10.4085/1062-6050-90-17.

Lepage, Christian, Marc Muehlmann, Yorghos Tripodis, Jakob Hufschmidt, Julie Stamm, Katie Green, Pawel Wrobel, et al. "Limbic System Structure Volumes and Associated Neurocognitive Functioning in Former NFL Players." *Brain Imaging and Behavior* 13, no. 3 (2018): 725–34. https://doi.org/10.1007/s11682-018-9895-z.

Lerner, Alec, and Norman Fost. "Informed Consent for Youth Tackle Football: Implications of the AAP Policy Statement." *Pediatrics* 144, no. 5 (2019): e20191985. https://doi.org/10.1542/peds.2019-1985.

Lynall, Robert C., Landon B. Lempke, Rachel S. Johnson, Melissa N. Anderson, and Julianne D. Schmidt. "A Comparison of Youth Flag and Tackle Football Head Impact Biomechanics." *Journal of Neurotrauma* 36 (2019): 1752–57. https://doi.org/10.1089/neu.2018.6236.

Malina, Robert M., Peter J. Morano, Mary Barron, Susan J. Miller, Sean P. Cumming, Anthony P. Kontos, and Bertis B. Little. "Overweight and Obesity among Youth Participants in American Football." *Journal of Pediatrics* 151, no. 4 (2007): 378–82. https://doi.org/10.1016/j.jpeds.2007.03.044.

Martini, Douglas, James Eckner, Jeffrey Kutcher, and Steven P. Broglio. "Subconcussive Head Impact Biomechanics: Comparing Differing Offensive Schemes." *Medicine & Science in Sports & Exercise* 45, no. 4 (2013): 755–61. https://doi.org/10.1249/MSS.0b013e3182798758.

McCrea, Michael, Steven Broglio, Thomas Mcallister, Wenxian Zhou, Shi Zhao, Barry Katz, Maria Kudela, et al. "Return to Play and Risk of Repeat Concussion in Collegiate Football Players: Comparative Analysis from the NCAA Concussion Study (1999–2001) and CARE Consortium (2014–2017)." *British Journal of Sports Medicine* 54, no. 2 (2019): 102–9. https://doi.org/10.1136/bjsports-2019-100579.

McGuine, Timothy, Eric Post, Adam Yakuro Pfaller, Scott Hetzel, Allison Schwarz, M. Alison Brooks, and Stephanie A. Kliethermes. "Does Soccer Headgear Reduce the Incidence of Sport-Related Concussion? A Cluster, Randomised Controlled Trial of Adolescent Athletes." *British Journal of Sports Medicine* 54, no. 7 (2020): 408–13. https://doi.org/10.1136/bjsports-2018-100238.

McKee, Ann C., Nigel J. Cairns, Dennis W. Dickson, Rebecca D. Folkerth, C. Dirk Keene, Irene Litvan, Daniel P. Perl, et al. "The First NINDS/NIBIB Consensus Meeting to Define Neuropathological Criteria for the Diagnosis of Chronic Traumatic Encephalopathy." *Acta Neuropathologica* 131, no. 1 (2016): 75–86. https://doi.org/10.1007/s00401-015-1515-z.

McKee, Ann C., Robert C. Cantu, Christopher J. Nowinski, E. Tessa Hedley-Whyte, Brandon E. Gavett, Andrew E. Budson, Veronica E. Santini, et al. "Chronic Traumatic Encephalopathy in Athletes: Progressive Tauopathy after Repetitive Head Injury." *Journal of Neuropathology and Experimental Neurology* 68, no. 7 (2009): 709–35. https://doi.org/10.1097/NEN.0b013e3181a9d503.

McKee, Ann C., Thor D. Stein, Christopher J. Nowinski, Robert A. Stern, Daniel H. Daneshvar, Victor E. Alvarez, Hyo-soon Lee, et al. "The Spectrum of Disease in Chronic Traumatic Encephalopathy." *Brain* 136 (2013): 43–64. https://doi.org/10.1093/brain/aws307.

McLaughlin, Katie A., David Weissman, and Debbie Bitrán. "Childhood Adversity and Neural Development: A Systematic Review." *Annual Review of Developmental Psychology* 1 (2019): 277–312. https://doi.org/10.1146/annurev-devpsych-121318-084950.

Mez, Jesse, Daniel H. Daneshvar, Bobak Abdolmohammadi, Alicia S. Chua, Michael L. Alosco, Patrick T. Kiernan, Laney Evers, et al. "Duration of American Football Play and Chronic Traumatic Encephalopathy." *Annals of Neurology* 87, no. 1 (2020): 116–31. https://doi.org/10.1002/ana.25611.

Mez, Jesse, Daniel H. Daneshvar, Patrick T. Kiernan, Bobak Abdolmohammadi, Victor E. Alvarez, Bertrand R. Huber, Michael L. Alosco, et al. "Clinicopathological Evaluation of Chronic Traumatic Encephalopathy in Players of American Football." *JAMA* 318, no. 4 (2017): 360–70. https://doi.org/10.1001/jama.2017.8334.

Mihalik, Jason P., David R. Bell, Stephen W. Marshall, and Kevin M. Guskiewicz. "Measurement of Head Impacts in Collegiate Football Players: An Investigation of Positional and Event-Type Differences." *Neurosurgery* 61, no. 6 (2007): 1229–35. https://doi.org/10.1227/01.neu.0000306103.68635.1a.

Mihalik, Jason P., Richard M. Greenwald, J. Troy Blackburn, Robert C. Cantu, Stephen W. Marshall, and Kevin M. Guskiewicz. "Effect of Infraction Type on Head Impact Severity in Youth Ice Hockey." *Medicine & Science in Sports & Exercise* 42, no. 8 (2010): 1431–38. https://doi.org/10.1249/MSS.0b013e3181d2521a.

Mihalik, Jason P., Kevin M. Guskiewicz, Stephen W. Marshall, Richard M. Greenwald, J. Troy Blackburn, and Robert C. Cantu. "Does Cervical Muscle Strength in Youth Ice Hockey Players Affect Head Impact Biomechanics?" *Clinical Journal of Sport Medicine* 21, no. 5 (2011): 416–21. https://doi.org/10.1097/JSM.0B013E31822C8A5C.

Mihalik, Jason P., Erin B. Wasserman, Elizabeth F. Teel, and Stephen W. Marshall. "Head Impact Biomechanics Differ between Girls and Boys Youth Ice Hockey Players." *Annals of Biomedical Engineering* 48, no. 1 (2019): 104–11. https://doi.org/10.1007/s10439-019-02343-9.

Miles, Steven H., and Shailendra Prasad. "Medical Ethics and School Football." *American Journal of Bioethics* 16, no. 1 (2016): 6–10. https://doi.org/10.1080/15265161.2016.1128751.

Montenigro, Philip H., Michael L. Alosco, Brett M. Martin, Daniel H. Daneshvar, Jesse Mez, Christine E. Chaisson, Christopher J. Nowinski, et al. "Cumulative Head Impact Exposure Predicts Later-Life Depression, Apathy, Executive Dysfunction, and Cognitive Impairment in Former High School and College Football Players." *Journal of Neurotrauma* 34 (2017): 328–40. https://doi.org/10.1089/neu.2016.4413.

Munce, Thayne A., Jason C. Dorman, Paul A. Thompson, Verle D. Valentine, and Michael F. Bergeron. "Head Impact Exposure and Neurologic Function of Youth Football Players." *Medicine & Science in Sports & Exercise* 47, no. 8 (2015): 1567–76. https://doi.org/10.1249/MSS.0000000000000591.

Narayana, Shalini, Christopher Charles, Kassondra Collins, Jack W. Tsao, Ansley Grimes Stanfill, and Brandon Baughman. "Neuroimaging and Neuropsychological Studies in Sports-Related Concussions in Adolescents: Current State and Future Directions." *Frontiers in Neurology* 10 (2019): 1–10. https://doi.org/10.3389/fneur.2019.00538.

O'Connor, Kathryn L., Steven Rowson, Stefan M. Duma, and Steven P. Broglio. "Head-Impact–Measurement Devices: A Systematic Review." *Journal of Athletic Training* 52, no. 3 (2017): 206–27. https://doi.org/10.4085/1062-6050.52.2.05.

O'Kane, John W., Amy Spieker, Marni R. Levy, Moni Neradilek, Nayak L. Polissar, and Melissa A. Schiff. "Concussion among Female Middle-School Soccer Players." *JAMA Pediatrics* 168, no. 3 (2019): 258–64. https://doi.org/10.1001/jamapediatrics.2013.4518.

Peterson, Andrew R., Adam J. Kruse, Scott M. Meester, Tyler S. Olson, Benjamin N. Riedle, Tyler G. Slayman, Todd J. Domeyer, et al. "Youth Football Injuries: A Prospective Cohort." *Orthopaedic Journal of Sports Medicine* 5, no. 2 (2017). https://doi.org/10.1177/2325967116686784.

Pfaller, Adam Y., M. Alison Brooks, Scott Hetzel, and Timothy A. McGuine. "Effect of a New Rule Limiting Full Contact Practice on the Incidence of Sport-Related Concussion in High School Football Players." *American Journal of Sports Medicine* 47, no. 10 (2019): 2294–99. https://doi.org/10.1177/0363546519860120.

Press, Jaclyn N., and Steven Rowson. "Quantifying Head Impact Exposure in Collegiate Women's Soccer." *Clinical Journal of Sport Medicine* 27 (2017): 104–10. https://doi.org/10.1097/JSM.0000000000000313.

Reed, N., M. Keightley, J. McAuliffe, J. Cubos, J. Baker, B. Faught, M. McPherson, et al. "Measurement of Head Impacts in Youth Ice Hockey Players." *Orthopedics & Biomechanics* 31 (2010): 826–33. https://doi.org/10.1055/s-0030-1263103.

Register-Mihalik, Johna K., Richelle M. Williams, Stephen W. Marshall, Laura A. Linnan, Jason P. Mihalik, Kevin M. Guskiewicz, and Tamara C. Valovich McLeod. "Demographic, Parental, and Personal Factors and Youth Athletes' Concussion-Related Knowledge and Beliefs." *Journal of Athletic Training* 53, no. 8 (2018): 768–75. https://doi.org/10.4085/1062-6050-223-17.

Robbins, Clifford A., Daniel H. Daneshvar, John D. Picano, Brandon E. Gavett, Christine M. Baugh, David O. Riley, Christopher J. Nowinski, et al. "Self-Reported Concussion History: Impact of Providing a Definition of Concussion." *Open Access Journal of Sports Medicine* 5 (2014): 99–103. https://doi.org/10.2147/OAJSM.S58005.

Rowson, Steven, Eamon T. Campolettano, Stefan M. Duma, Brian Stemper, Alok Shah, Jaroslaw Harezlak, Larry Riggen, et al. "Accounting for Variance in Concussion Tolerance between Individuals: Comparing Head Accelerations between Concussed and Physically Matched Control Subjects." *Annals of Biomedical Engineering* 47, no. 10 (2019): 2048–56. https://doi.org/10.1007/s10439-019-02329-7.

Sarmiento, Kelly, Zoe Donnell, and Rosanne Hoffman. "A Scooping Review to Address the Culture of Concussion in Youth and High School Sports." *School Health* 87, no. 10 (2017): 790–804. https://doi.org/10.1111/josh.12552.

Sarmiento, Kelly, Karen E. Thomas, Jill Daugherty, Dana Waltzman, Juliet K. Haarbauer-Krupa, Alexis B. Peterson, Tadesse Haileyesus, et al. "Emergency Department Visits for Sports- and Recreation-Related Traumatic Brain Injuries among Children—United States, 2010–2016." *Centers for Disease Control Morbidity and Mortality Weekly Report* 68, no. 10 (2019): 237–42. https://doi.org/10.15585/mmwr.mm6810a2.

Schmidt, Julianne D., Alice F. Pierce, Kevin M. Guskiewicz, Johna K. Register-Mihalik, Derek N. Pamukoff, and Jason P. Mihalik. "Safe-Play Knowledge, Aggression, and Head-Impact Biomechanics in Adolescent Ice Hockey Players." *Journal of Athletic Training* 51, no. 5 (2016): 366–72. https://doi.org/10.4085/1062-6050-51.5.04.

Schultz, Vivian, Robert A. Stern, Yorghos Tripodis, Julie Stamm, Pawel Wrobel, Christian Lepage, Isabelle Weir, et al. "Age at First Exposure to Repetitive Head Impacts Is Associated with Smaller Thalamic Volumes in Former Professional American Football Players." *Journal of Neurotrauma* 35, no. 2 (2017): 278–85. https://doi.org/10.1089/neu.2017.5145.

Schwarz, Alan. "N.F.L.-Backed Youth Program Says It Reduced Concussions. The Data Disagrees." *New York Times*, July 27, 2016. https://www.nytimes.com/2016/07/28/sports/football/nfl-concussions-youth-program-heads-up-football.html.

Seichepine, Daniel R., Julie M. Stamm, Daniel H. Daneshvar, David O. Riley, Christine M. Baugh, Brandon E. Gavett, Yorghos Tripodis, et al. "Profile of Self-Reported Problems with Executive Functioning in College and Professional Football Players." *Journal of Neurotrauma* 30, no. 14 (2013): 1299–1304. https://doi.org/10.1089/neu.2012.2690.

Shankman, Sabrina. "Report Warned Riddell about Helmets." ESPN, April 30, 2013. https://www.espn.com/espn/otl/story/_/id/9228260/report-warned-riddell-no-helmet-prevent-concussions-nfl-helmet-maker-marketed-one-such-anyway.

Shrey, Daniel W., Grace S. Griesbach, and Christopher C. Giza. "The Pathophysiology of Concussions in Youth." *Physical Medicine & Rehabilitation Clinics of North America* 22, no. 4 (2012): 577–602. https://doi.org/10.1016/j.pmr.2011.08.002.

Siva, Nayanah. "Scotland to Ban Heading in Children's Football." *Lancet* 395, no. 10220 (2020): 258. https://doi.org/10.1016/S0140-6736(20)30118-5.

Skinner, Asheley Cockrell, Stephanie E. Hasty, Robert W. Turner II, Mark Dreibelbis, and Jacob A. Lohr. "Is Bigger Really Better? Obesity among High School Football Players, Player Position, and Team Success." *Clinical Pediatrics* 52, no. 10 (2013): 922–28. https://doi.org/10.1177/0009922813492880.

Small, Gary W., Vladimir Kepe, Prabha Siddarth, Linda M. Ercoli, David A. Merrill, Natacha Donoghue, Susan Y. Bookheimer, et al. "PET Scanning of Brain Tau in Retired National Football League Players: Preliminary Findings." *American Journal of Geriatric Psychiatry* 21, no. 2 (2013): 138–44. https://doi.org/10.1016/j.jagp.2012.11.019.

Smith, Aynsley M., Michael J. Stuart, Daniel V. Gaz, Casey P. Twardowski, Michael B. Stuart, David Margeneau, Hal Tearse, et al. "Behavioral Modification to Reduce Concussion in Collision Sports: Ice Hockey." *Current Sports Medicine Reports* 12, no. 6 (2013): 3–6. https://doi.org/10.1249/JSR.0000000000000004.

Snook, Lindsay, Lori-Anne Paulson, Dawne Roy, Linda Phillips, and Christian Beaulieu. "Diffusion Tensor Imaging of Neurodevelopment in Children and Young Adults." *NeuroImage* 26, no. 4 (2005): 1164–73. https://doi.org/10.1016/j.neuroimage.2005.03.016.

Solomon, Gary S., Andrew W. Kuhn, Scott L. Zuckerman, Ira R. Casson, David C. Viano, Mark R. Lovell, and Allen K. Sills. "Participation in Pre–High School Football and Neurological, Neuroradiological, and Neuropsychological Findings in Later Life: A Study of 45 Retired National Football League Players." *American Journal of Sports Medicine* 44, no. 5 (2016): 1106–15. https://doi.org/10.1177/0363546 515626164.

Stamm, Julie M., Alexandra P. Bourlas, Christine M. Baugh, Nathan G. Fritts, Daniel H. Daneshvar, Brett M. Martin, Michael D. McClean, et al. "Age of First Exposure to Football and Later-Life Cognitive Impairment in Former NFL Players." *Neurology* 84, no. 11 (2015): 1114–20. https://doi.org/10.1212/WNL.0000000000001358.

Stamm, Julie M., Inga K. Koerte, Marc Muehlmann, Ofer Pasternak, Alexandra P. Bourlas, Christine M. Baugh, Michelle Y. Giwerc, et al. "Age at First Exposure to Football Is Associated with Altered Corpus Callosum White Matter Microstructure in Former Professional Football Players." *Journal of Neurotrauma* 32 (2015): 1768–76. https://doi.org/10.1089/neu.2014.3822.

Stamm, Julie M., Eric G. Post, Christine M. Baugh, and David R. Bell. "Awareness of Concussion Education Requirements, Management Plans, and Knowledge in High School and Club Sport Coaches." *Journal of Athletic Training* 55, no. 10 (2020): 1054–61. https://doi.org/10.4085/1062-6050-0394-19.

Stemper, Brian D., Alok S. Shah, Jaroslaw Harezlak, Steven Rowson, Stefan Duma, Jason P. Mihalik, Larry D. Riggen, et al. "Repetitive Head Impact Exposure in College Football following an NCAA Rule Change to Eliminate Two-a-Day Preseason Practices: A Study from the NCAA-DoD CARE Consortium." *Annals of Biomedical Engineering* 47, no. 10 (2019): 2073–85. https://doi.org/10.1007/s10439-019-02335-9.

Stemper, Brian D., Alok S. Shah, Jaroslaw Harezlak, Steven Rowson, Jason P. Mihalik, Stefan Duma, Larry D. Riggen, et al. "Comparison of Head Impact Exposure between Concussed Football Athletes and Matched Controls: Evidence for a Possible Second Mechanism of Sport-Related Concussion." *Annals of Biomedical Engineering* 47, no. 10 (2018): 2057–72. https://doi.org/10.1007/s10439-018-02136-6.

Stemper, Brian D., Alok S. Shah, Jason P. Mihalik, Jaroslaw Harezlak, Steven Rowson, Stefan Duma, Larry D. Riggen, et al. "Head Impact Exposure in College Football following a Reduction in Preseason Practices." *Medicine & Science in Sports & Exercise* 52, no. 7 (2020): 1629–38. https://doi.org/10.1249/MSS.0000000000002283.

Stern, Robert A., Daniel H. Daneshvar, Christine M. Baugh, Daniel R. Seichepine, Phillip H. Montenigro, David O. Riley, Nathan G. Fritts, et al. "Clinical Presentation of Chronic Traumatic Encephalopathy." *Neurology* 81 (2013): 1122–29. https://doi.org/10.1212/WNL.0b013e3182a55f7f.

Stokes, Keith A., Duncan Locke, Simon Roberts, Lewis Henderson, Ross Tucker, Dean Ryan, and Simon Kemp. "Does Reducing the Height of the Tackle through Law Change in Elite Men's Rugby Union (The Championship, England) Reduce the Incidence of Concussion? A Controlled Study in 126 Games." *British Journal of Sports Medicine* (2019): 1–6. https://doi.org/10.1136/bjsports-2019-101557.

Svaldi, Diana O., Emily C. McCuen, Chetas Joshi, Meghan E. Robinson, Yeseul Nho, Robert Hannemann, Eric A. Nauman, et al. "Cerebrovascular Reactivity Changes in Asymptomatic Female Athletes Attributable to High School Soccer Participation." *Brain Imaging and Behavior* 11 (2017): 98–112. https://doi.org/10.1007/s11682-016-9509-6.

Swartz, Erik E., Jay L. Myers, Summer B. Cook, Kevin M. Guskiewicz, Michael S. Ferrara, Robert C. Cantu, Hong Chang, et al. "A Helmetless-Tackling Intervention in American Football for Decreasing Head Impact Exposure: A Randomized Controlled Trial." *Journal of Science and Medicine in Sport* 22, no. 10 (2019): 1102–7. https://doi.org/10.1016/j.jsams.2019.05.018.

Uematsu, Akiko, Mie Matsui, Chiaki Tanaka, Tsutomu Takahashi, Kyo Noguchi, Michio Suzuki, and Hisao Nishijo. "Developmental Trajectories of Amygdala and Hippocampus from Infancy to Early Adulthood in Healthy Individuals." *PLOS ONE* 7, no. 10 (2012): e46970. https://doi.org/10.1371/journal.pone.0046970.

USA Hockey. "Hockey in the United States: A Growing Game." November 8, 2018. https://www.usahockey.com/news_article/show/966542.

"Virginia Tech Helmet Ratings." https://helmet.beam.vt.edu/index.html. Accessed June 14, 2020.

Wallace, Jessica, Tracey Covassin, and Erica Beidler. "Sex Differences in High School Athletes' Knowledge of Sport-Related Concussion Symptoms and Reporting Behaviors." *Journal of Athletic Training* 52, no. 7 (2017): 682–88. https://doi.org/10.4085/1062-6050-52.3.06.

Wilcox, Bethany J., Jonathan G. Beckwith, Richard M. Greenwald, Jeffrey J. Chu, Thomas W. McAllister, Laura A. Flashman, Arthur C. Maerlender, et al. "Head Impact Exposure in Male and Female Collegiate Ice Hockey Players." *Journal of Biomechanics* 47 (2014): 109–14. https://doi.org/10.1016/j.jbiomech.2013.10.004.

Young, Tyler J., Ray W. Daniel, Steven Rowson, and Stefan M. Duma. "Head Impact Exposure in Youth Football: Elementary School Ages 7-8 Years and the Effect of Returning Players." *Clinical Journal of Sport Medicine* 24, no. 4 (2014): 416–21. https://doi.org/10.1097/JSM.0000000000000055.

Zuckerman, Scott L., Zachary Y. Kerr, Aaron Yengo-Kahn, Erin Wasserman, Tracey Covassin, and Gary S. Solomon. "Epidemiology of Sports-Related Concussion in NCAA Athletes from 2009–2010 to 2013–2014." *American Journal of Sports Medicine* 43, no. 11 (2015): 2654–62. https://doi.org/10.1177/0363546515599634.

Index

225

About the Author

Julie M. Stamm has spent a decade studying concussions and the long-term consequences of repetitive brain trauma in sports, with a focus on how that trauma impacts brain development. She earned her doctorate in anatomy and neurobiology from the Boston University School of Medicine and conducted research at the Boston University Chronic Traumatic Encephalopathy Center and the Psychiatry Neuroimaging Laboratory at Harvard Medical School, Brigham and Women's Hospital. She is a proud alumna of the University of Wisconsin–Madison, where she earned her degree in kinesiology/athletic training. She is a certified athletic trainer with experience providing medical care for athletes at the high school and college levels. Stamm is currently a clinical assistant professor at the University of Wisconsin–Madison.

CPSIA information can be obtained
at www.ICGtesting.com
Printed in the USA
LVHW091521140721
692682LV00001B/75